THE MARTIAL ARTS ATHLETE

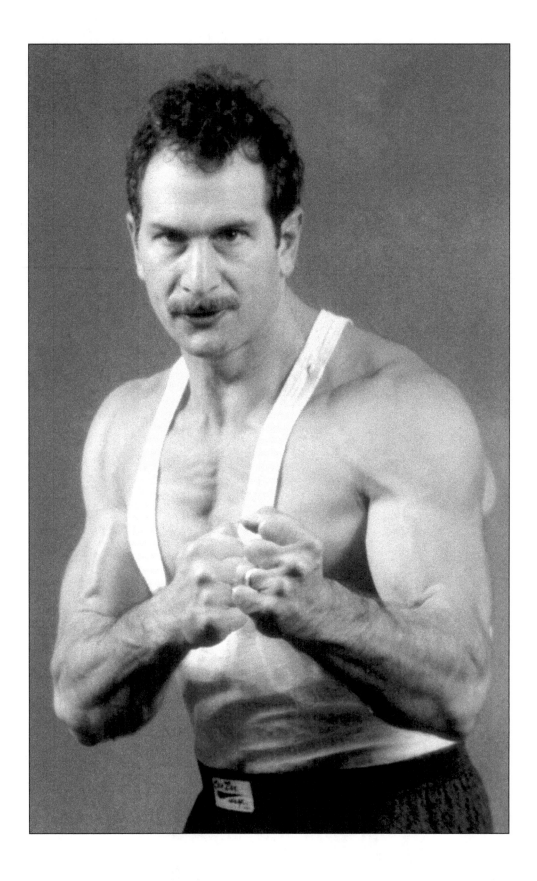

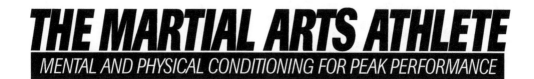

THE MARTIAL ARTS ATHLETE
MENTAL AND PHYSICAL CONDITIONING FOR PEAK PERFORMANCE

Tom Seabourne, Ph.D.

YMAA Publication Center
Wolfeboro, NH USA

YMAA Publication Center
Main Office
 PO Box 480
 Wolfeboro, NH 02131 USA
 1-800-669-8892 • www.ymaa.com • info@ymaa.com

20200403

ISBN-13: 978159439650 • ISBN-10:1886969655

Publisher's Cataloging in Publication
(Prepared by Quality Books Inc.)

Seabourne, Thomas.
 The martial arts athlete : mental and physical conditioning
for peak performance / Tom Seabourne. — 1st ed.
 p. cm. —(Martial arts—external)
 ISBN: 1-886969-65-5

 1. Martial arts—Training.   I. Title. II. Series

GV1102.7.T7S43 1998   796.8
                             QBI98-736

Photographs by Ron Barker

Cover design by Richard Rossiter

Figures 2-1, 2-7, 2-8, 2-9, 2-10, 2-12, 2-74, 5-1, 5-4, 5-7, 5-10, 5-21, and 5-45 copyright
©1994 by TechPool Studios Corp. USA, 1463 Warrensville Center Road, Cleveland, OH 44121.

Disclaimer:
The authors and publisher of this material are NOT RESPONSIBLE in any manner whatso-
ever for any injury which may occur through reading or following the instructions in this
manual.
The activities, physical or otherwise, described in this material may be too strenuous or
dangerous for some people, and the reader(s) should consult a physician before engaging in
them.

Printed in USA.

Table of Contents

1.1 The Present is Rooted in the Past
1.2 How to Use This Book
1.3 Individual Choice

2.1 Awesome Abdominals
2.2 A Strong Back
2.3 Jumping Rope
2.4 Incredible Flexibility
2.5 Isometric Stances
2.6 Plyometrics for Explosive Power
2.7 Form Training
2.8 Balance

3.1 Everything Begins in Your Mind
3.2 Focus
3.3 Self Talk
3.4 Pain Management
3.5 Rhythm
3.6 Discipline
3.7 Burning Desire
3.8 Overtraining

4.1 Breathing
4.2 Relaxation
4.3 Meditation
4.4 Imagery
4.5 Mind and Body

5.1 Training Anytime, Anywhere!
5.2 Training Solo
5.3 Strength Training
5.4 Using Dumbbells
5.5 Mind Over Muscle
5.6 If You Don't Have Weights
5.7 Cross-Martial Arts Training
5.8 Team Training
5.9 Nutrition for Peak Performance

6.1 Putting It All Together
6.2 Ten Tips to Master Your Art

Acknowledgements

I would like to dedicate this book to the memory of my father Thomas G. Seabourne who inspired my travels to China, Japan, and Europe to study and compete with the most formidable martial artists in the world.

Thanks to my mother Ann, my wife Danese, my daughters, Alaina, Laura, Susanna, and Julia, and my son, Grant for allowing me to share with them my love for the martial arts.

Thanks also to Tandi Joleen Holloway and Monica Norfleet for their appearances in many of the photographs found in this book, and a special thank you to YMAA for helping me gather my thoughts into a readable text.

Foreword

I met Tom Seabourne at the Taekwondo World Cup in Colorado Springs in 1986. He was the sports psychologist/physiologist for the U.S. Team. I was having trouble sleeping the night before my bouts and it really concerned me.

The pressure was unrelenting. I asked Tom what to do. His reply was, "Herb, it's not the amount of sleep that you get the night before your fight, it's the quality of sleep you get the WEEKS before." He was right! I know that I had been getting pretty good sleep before the events and the more I thought about what Tom said, the more it made sense. The pressure was off! I was ready! With that advice and using some of Tom's techniques I was able to win gold medals at the World Cup, Pan Am games, and finally at the 1992 Olympic Games in Barcelona

Martial artists today are looking for more than just self-defense techniques. We are training for improved health, better body fitness, clarity of mind and of course, competition. The trouble is that you probably can't attain all of these goals training only during class time at your school.

Dr. Tom Seabourne's book *The Martial Arts Athlete* takes the guesswork out of training. As a two-time member of the U.S. Taekwondo Team and Silver Medalist in the World Championships, Tom knows what it is like to compete at an elite level. But more than that, Dr. Seabourne has spent years studying physiology and psychology so that he provides you with the science for your success, but without the hard to understand jargon.

This is the same method that Tom provided to me in my early years of competition, and now it is available to all by virtue of his new book. Tom is one of the few elite athlete-scholars who has joined an even fewer elite producers of training material for martial artists. His books are on the shelves of every serious martial artist around the world.

I have trained and traveled around the world with Taekwondo. I don't think a minute goes by without thinking about my love for this art. Whether you aspire to become an Olympian, or if you just want to be your best, I highly recommend that you read *The Martial Arts Athlete—Mental and Physical Conditioning for Peak Performance.*

Herb Perez
1992 Olympic Gold Medalist
Taekwondo

Preface

In junior high I was an MVP football player until I dropped a game-winning touchdown pass. My teammates forgave me but I never forgave my "Charlie Brown choke." I haven't played team sports since. Instead, at thirteen I quit football and focused on martial arts. Disciplined practice was my passion. My solitary workouts were emotional. My buddies thought I was nuts. I remember New Year's Eve, sneaking past my parents' guests down to my musty basement, practicing martial arts drills until my clothes were soaked.

My master once commented, "Make your feet like your hands." From then on my combination kicks blossomed. My front leg double roundhouse kick resembles a boxer's double jab. And my rear leg side kick can be likened to a right cross. My front leg hook kick looks like a boxer's hook. And my rear leg front kick favors an uppercut.

Many people feel they cannot do their best because they have not learned the Far Eastern concepts of discipline and self-control. It took me twenty years of studying Eastern philosophy and analyzing it in Western terms to develop and use a variety of mental preparations and physiological training techniques, to prepare me to win national and international martial arts events.

My study, training, and competition took place in Okinawa, Japan, China, and Europe, and encompassed traditional physiology, as well as a search for that elusive inner strength.

Understand that the psycho-physiological techniques in this book take practice, but whether you learn them from *The Martial Arts Athlete* or an aged wise man, the principles are essentially the same. These principles point the way to enhanced performance and wellness. Sometimes we must simply remind ourselves to use these secrets.

CHAPTER 1

The Martial Arts Athlete

1.1 The Present is Rooted in the Past

As an eleven year old kid growing up in Okinawa on a U.S. military base, my best buddy Ernest suggested we watch a martial arts class. We slipped over the barbed-wire fence separating the army base from the martial arts school situated in the ground floor of a hotel in an impoverished village. I was captivated with the discipline. Asians were attacking and defending in unison. The power in their technique was awesome. I convinced my dad that I deserved to be a student (Figure 1-1). Few Americans trained in our Asian martial arts school. Not because it cost six dollars per month. Nor was there a language barrier. For many Americans, doing the same program night after night, year after year, was boring. But not for me. When I looked at my front kick and compared it to my master's, I knew I had plenty to learn.

Most of us hung our uniforms on hangers in the locker room. There were no showers, and no female locker room. Showers would have made little difference because the humidity in the Far East was oppressive. Putting on a uniform felt like stepping into a cardboard box encrusted with hardened sweat. There was a placard in the training hall stating that uniforms must be laundered once a week. The day before I was to return to the United States, my master handed me a pin and said, "Never change styles."

Several students, like myself, returned to the United States and opened branch schools. Upon my family's return to Pennsylvania, I

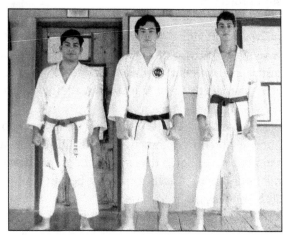

Fig 1-1

1

was frustrated that there were no martial arts studios. I trained by myself daily for two years until a martial arts school opened a mile from my home.

My parents hoped I would play football as a youngster, but I chose to practice martial arts instead. At first it appeared to be a bad decision. I was tall, thin, and could never keep my balance. My instructor kicked my unstable stance out from under me, knocking me to the floor. I trained harder and more often than my fellow classmates, sometimes four hours a day. When my master visited the United States ten years later, he was amazed to see me in the finals of a national championship. He watched me reach my goal in an art that has been a passion for me since he taught me my first lesson.

I ate, slept, and drank martial arts, competing in Asia and Europe against some of the best fighters in the world (Figure 1-2). I learned that there are three traits champion martial artists possess:

1. They love their art.
2. They are in great shape.
3. They master one, maybe two strikes or kicks.

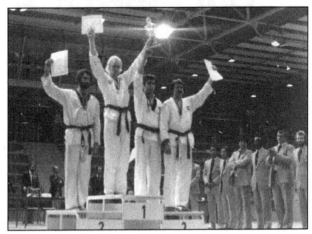

Fig 1-2

1.2 How to Use This Book

In the old days we sparred without pads. Our forearms and shins were bruised. Rather than protect ourselves, we practiced pounding each other's limbs to toughen them. Today I can run my fingers up and down my shins and forearms and find calcium deposits. Twenty years later, I demand my students use forearm pads and shin protectors.

I, like most of you, no longer have the time to devote every minute of every day to martial arts training. This book is a guide to maximizing the training time you do have. Each practice session is a work of art. The palette is your body and mind. And just as in a work of art, when the elements are used correctly, the effects are indescribable. Martial arts training is the best thing you can do for your body/mind, and your body/mind can do for you.

You can practice the techniques in this book, both physical and mental, at your preferred intensity. It is better to train three times a week for twenty minutes than to train two hours, seven days a week for a month, and then quit. This book allows you the flexibility to pick the skills that best fit your physique and personality, and to find areas you most want to develop.

The Martial Arts Athlete is designed for students of all martial arts styles and is compatible with any system. It does not teach you a martial arts 'style'. Instead, this book offers you proven training techniques that you can apply to whatever martial art you are learning to help you achieve your very best.

The Martial Arts Athlete contains workouts that are both mentally and physically tough. But don't look at the photos and say, "I can't do that." If you truly can't do it, then you need to learn. Peruse this book and find an area that interests you. Pick any one of the program objectives and follow the instructions. The more you practice, the better your results. Do not attempt to modify more than one set of behaviors at a time. Speed, power, and eating correctly are important. However, quieting your mind and developing a sense of inner peace are just as valuable.

Some of the benefits you will gain from regular practice of the techniques in this book include: increased flexibility, injury prevention, better body alignment, less stress, better concentration, greater endurance, increased fighting ability, increased strength, decreased body fat, and improved confidence. This is a holistic program designed to make you the best martial artist you can be.

1.3 Individual Choice

Each evening Ernest and I trained with my classmates under the watchful eye of our master. I was tall for my age, skinny, clumsy, and a slow learner. The teacher was unimpressed with my ability. We did an identical program six nights a week. Two weeks after we joined, Ernest decided to play basketball instead. I made the pilgrimage nightly, alone. In summers, I attended both morning and evening sessions. I trained before and after class to offset my lack of ability. Rather than watch television, I punched and kicked alone in my basement.

In martial arts, you must make the choice to give up some of your less important activities. Awareness of your goals and aspirations is the first step. Surround yourself with people who will encourage you. From morning until bedtime, we are so busy that we rarely take time to identify our mission in life. If your mission comes from within, motivation will be easy.

I cannot tell you what purpose to strive for, but maybe I can inspire you to start searching. When you are ready, you will start. It is your level of readiness that determines your motivation. When you are motivated, you will begin.

After you decide on a martial arts goal, figure out why you want to do it. Then decide how you will get there. And finally, imagine what you will do when you get there. Know specifically what you are attempting to achieve. Set short and long term targets. Establish both martial arts objectives and outcome goals. Resist the temptation to compare your performance with others. To reach your highest levels, compete with yourself.

Goal setting is the aim or purpose of an action. It provides direction and guides you on your martial arts journey. Goals direct your attention toward accomplishing a task. Accomplishment that increases your self-esteem is not just about doing something. It is about the courage to persist through pain, failure, and self-doubt.

Some martial artists seem to have an inner drive to succeed. It appears inborn. But the truth is that persistent, unyielding effort makes it happen. We are not born with mental toughness. It must be trained and practiced. The ability to manage adversity, relax under pressure, and maintain a goal-directed focus are not magically learned. You must direct your thoughts and emotions. Then you can maintain a high level of concentration from day to day.

Initially, speed and power are not pertinent to your martial arts; step through the motions emphasizing precision. Later, you can focus on details, including the position of your feet, knees, toes, and upper body. As you persist in your training, create techniques that work best for your body structure, personality, and the demands of each circumstance. Rather than mindlessly rehearsing hundreds of different attacks, select a few and hone them into personalized weapons.

Sample Outline of Your Training Schedule

1. Begin each workout with an abdominal warm up. Contract your muscles when you feel a slight bit of pressure. Hold that tension, then relax.
2. Following your abdominal routine, jump rope for five minutes.
3. After jumping rope, move on to stretching. When you execute each stretch, hold it for a few seconds, then relax. As you advance, add two seconds each week until you are holding each posture for thirty seconds.
4. After stretching, practice your punches, kicks, strikes, blocks, and footwork. Devoting time to these fundamentals broadens your foundation. Advanced techniques have their roots in beginning level moves. A side hook kick cannot be done effectively without perfecting the side snap kick. A flying spinning back kick may look impossible at first. But it can be thrown effortlessly if the basics have been mastered. Build upon your elementary techniques until you master your art.

CHAPTER 2

Mastering the Basics: Strength, Speed, Flexibility, Power

2.1 Awesome Abdominals

Training overseas, we did no abdominal exercise. Our paunches got a decent workout from two hours of kicks, punches, strikes and blocks. For example, put this book down and punch with your right hand while you exhale. Place your left hand lightly over your stomach and punch-exhale again. You should be able to feel your abdominals contract.

Why Train Abdominal Muscles?

Most athletes concentrate on strengthening their bodies depending on their sport. For example, sprinters work on their legs. But if they do not train their upper bodies they will not run as fast. Similarly, as a martial artist, although you concentrate on your arms and legs, you cannot ignore your abdominals.

Although your abs do not appear to be directly involved in martial arts, they are. You can move with increased balance and body control if your midsection is strong enough to steady your movement. Improving strength in your abs will help you change directions. You can lift twice as much weight. Your back won't get sore after you work out. And you can take a shot to the body that would make most people cringe.

The center of your body is the place where your power begins. Martial artists have known this for centuries. You focus your '*chi*' from a place two inches below your navel. If you are centered, you will increase your energy and power. A powerful midline provides a base so you may explode through your punches. Whether you do kicks or throws, force is generated from your midsection. If your abs are weak, your power chain is broken.

Your torso is a vital area for you to tone and strengthen to increase your power. Torso exercises stabilize the spine and protect you from injury. Abdominal muscles allow your torso to turn, twist, and bend so you can remain comfortable in the ring. Your waist connects your upper and lower body to generate the tremendous torque necessary for dynamic punching and kicking.

A strong middle connects your upper and lower body. The muscles in the front and side of your belly help raise your legs to execute all of your kicks. The muscles that run diagonally across your ribs and those that sit above them help keep your posture. A strong midline prevents injury. Strong stomach muscles also protect your internal organs.

A strong abdomen stabilizes motion for peak efficiency. Your abdominals must stabilize your torso. When practicing or sparring, your center of gravity constantly changes. For example, your center of gravity is outside of your body during a flying side kick. Your center of gravity lowers when you bend your knees to deliver a commanding punch. Therefore you should prepare your torso for flexion (leaning forward), extension (leaning backward), and rotation (turning sideways) by training your abs and obliques. You can move at a variety of angles and feel secure if your abs are trained.

Finally, if you are striving to develop a lean look and a washboard stomach, abdominal exercises will tone and strengthen the muscles.

The Six Pack and Other Abs

The set of abdominal muscles referred to as the 'six pack' are your rectus abdominis (Figure 2-1). And in reality they are a 'ten pack'. The origin of this muscle group is your pubis bone. The insertion is located in the cartilage of ribs five through seven and your xiphoid process. The rectus abdominis is a strap-like muscle designed for smooth, long movement. Its main purpose is to raise your body from bed each morning. In order to train this muscle group, a simple crunch exercise is sufficient.

Beware of infomercial abdominal devices. Some train body parts which do not include your abs. To firm up your abs free of charge, lie on your back with your knees bent, and your chin resting on your chest (Figure 2-2). Tilt your pelvis until the small of your back begins to flatten to the floor (Figure 2-3). Curl your ribcage toward your

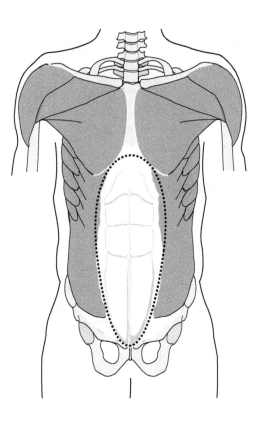

Fig 2-1. The 'Six Pack' (rectus abdominis)

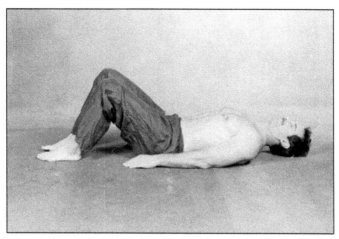

Fig 2-2

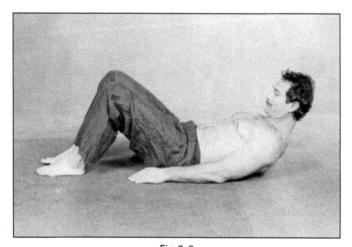

Fig 2-3

pelvis. Follow this progression: Tilt, curl, flex for two seconds, then untilt and uncurl. Focus on flexing your rectus abdominis. The range of motion is only a few inches. It feels as if you are working your upper abs because the top of your rectus abdominis is thinner than the layer towards the pubis. Perform ten repetitions. Use your rectus abdominis muscles to curl your body, not your head and neck.

To do a reverse crunch, lie on your back with your knees flexed to your chest. Place your hands under your hips (Figure 2-4). Keep your knees together as you bring your feet toward the floor (Figure 2-5). Hold for three seconds, then slowly draw your knees back to your chest (Figure 2-6). It feels as if you are working the lower part of your rectus abdominis because your hip flexor muscles (iliopsoas) (Figure 2-7) are assisting.

Two more sets of abdominal muscles are your external and internal obliques. Your external obliques are the "hands in your front pocket." The origin is on ribs five through twelve and the insertion is on the iliac crest and pubic bone (Figure 2-8). Your obliques are thin muscles. They are not designed for heavy resistance training. They

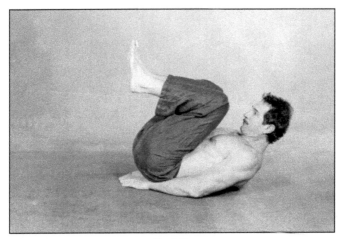

Fig 2-4

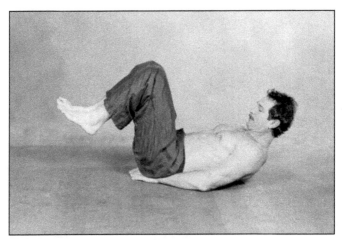

Fig 2-5

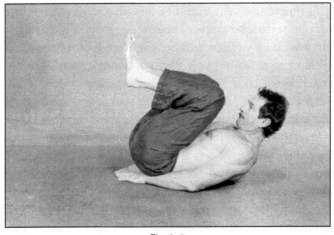

Fig 2-6

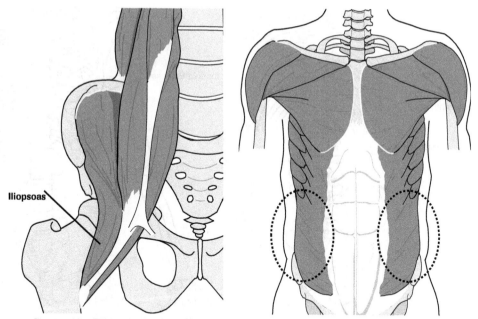

Fig 2-7. Hip Flexors (iliopsoas)   Fig 2-8. External and Internal Obliques

wrap around the torso enclosing the internal structures. Obliques act as protection and support; a suit of armor. These are the muscles you notice when you lift a heavy object. They protect your abdominal area during straining, sneezing, forced expiration, or bearing down. Strong obliques help to pull, lift, or push heavy objects. They steady the torso to keep gravity from pulling you out of a neutral position while standing or sitting. Your obliques help you to balance and move your pelvis and lower back. To train your obliques, follow the same technique as the crunch, except that you raise your upper body at an angle to the right or the left.

Your internal obliques are under your external obliques and surround your waist. Think of these as the "hands in your back pocket" muscles. They are shaped like an inverted V. Internal obliques stabilize your trunk. Your obliques are the only abdominal muscles constantly active during standing. They function while you are in an upright posture to brace your torso. The origin of the internal obliques is your iliac crest. They insert on ribs nine through twelve (Figure 2-9).

Another set of stabilizer muscles in your abdomen include your transversus abdominis. The origin of these muscles are the cartilage of the last six vertebrae, iliac crest, and lumbar fascia. The insertion is the xiphoid process and pubis (Figure 2-10). They run horizontally. Their primary purpose is to enable you to force an expiration such as a cough or sneeze.

Now that you understand the origin and insertion of the major muscle groups in your waist, you realize there is no isolating the 'upper' and 'lower' abs. Train your rectus abdominis with crunches, and your obliques with twists. Do other exercises for variety, but more is not always better. There is no magic to developing your core. Instead, it requires disciplined daily training. An Ab-Roller is fine, but you can obtain the same results from crunches.

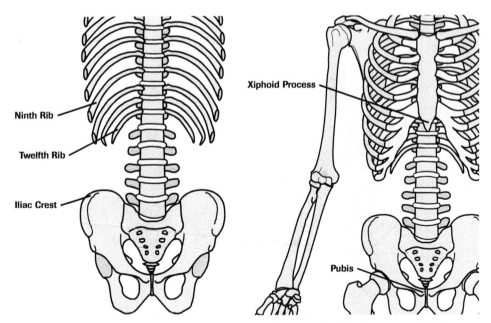

Fig 2-9. Muscle Attachments for Int. Obliques   Fig 2-10. Xiphoid Process and Pubis

To perform a perfect crunch, begin each repetition as if you were in slow motion. Contract your rectus abdominis and exhale as you let your muscles pull your shoulder blades off the floor. Exhaling on each repetition will allow you to squeeze your abs without arching your back. If crunches are too difficult, raise yourself off the floor with your arms and perform a crunch on the down phase.

An easy exercise to begin working your abs is pelvic tilts. Lie flat on your back and bend your knees keeping your feet flat on the floor. Extend your arms out to your side. Pull your abdominal muscles in and tighten your buttocks. Flatten the natural arch of your back against the floor (Figure 2-11). Hold your abdominals flexed for three seconds as you exhale. Then relax and take a deep breath. Do ten repetitions.

When you are attempting to train your abs, other, more powerful muscles called your hip flexors (iliopsoas) do most of the work. Even when you perform a crunch correctly, your rectus abdominis begins the movement but your hip flexors cannot help but become involved; especially if you attempt to perform crunches quickly. Raising slowly, and only coming up part way is your best method for working your rectus abdominis instead of your hip flexors.

If you anchor your feet, you work mostly hip flexors. With your feet anchored, your back may arch straining the quadratus laborum (lower back muscles) (Figure 2-12). Don't try twisting your elbow toward your knee at the top of your crunch. Instead, raise your elbow toward your opposite knee at the beginning of each repetition.

In my first martial arts tournament as a black belt, I was a freshman attending Pennsylvania State University. I found myself in the finals fighting for first place. Reaching the finals was thrilling, but I was matched against a tough opponent from Loyola College. My girlfriend was in the grandstands, and the center referee, Vance

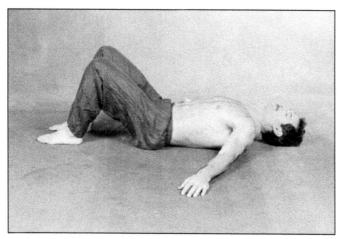

Fig 2-11

McLaughlin, was a karate hero of mine. I wanted to impress both of them. My high-kicking techniques scored heavily on my scrappy opponent.

In the final seconds of the last round, he caught me with a hard kick to my midsection. The force of the blow knocked the wind out of me, sending me doubled-over to the canvas. After writhing in pain a few moments, my hero, Mr. McLaughlin, pulled me up by my collar and commanded me to stand up straight. A time-out was called and I regained my composure for the final seconds of the match. Although I was declared the winner on points, it was a shallow victory. I was the one who was laid out on the mat. That match taught me the importance of strong abdominal muscles. Since then, I

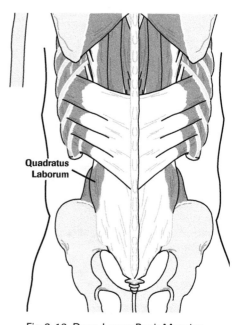

Fig 2-12. Deep Lower Back Muscles

have devoted ten minutes each day to my abdominal program as presented here and I have never been hurt by a blow to the midsection. You will strengthen muscles in your upper and lower stomach as well as your waist by following this program. Slowly curl up on all abdominal exercises. "Feel" the muscles working. Place your hands under your hips if you have a delicate back.

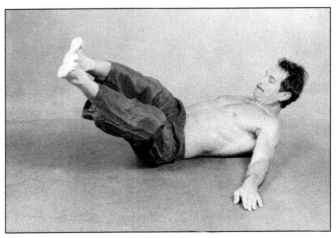

Fig 2-13

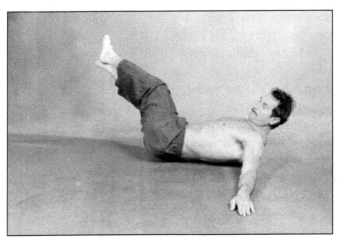

Fig 2-14

Abdominal Exercises

WARNING: On all of the exercises presented in this section, make sure to protect your back by keeping it flat to the floor or slightly arched.

Oblique Twists: This exercise works your lateral abdominals. Lie on your back with your arms out to the side, perpendicular to your body. Extend your legs up to a ninety degree angle with your knees slightly bent (Figure 2-13). Lower your legs to your right side so your feet barely touch the floor (Figure 2-14). Repeat, bringing your legs down to your left side. Alternate sides, doing ten repetitions each. Add two repetitions a week until you can perform twenty five repetitions on each side. This exercise strengthens your obliques.

V sit-ups: Support your back by propping your elbows behind you (Figure 2-15). Bring your knees to your chest and then extend your feet until your knees are just

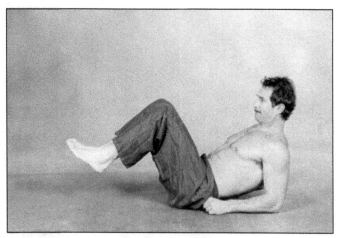

Fig 2-15

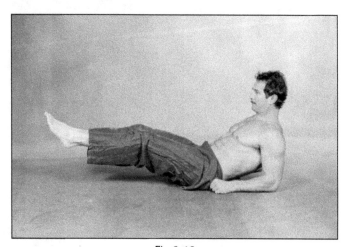

Fig 2-16

slightly bent (Figure 2-16). Repeat. This exercise develops strength in your rectus abdominis and hip flexors. If your back weakens and begins to arch, go to the next exercise.

Flutter kicks: Support your lower back by placing your elbows on the floor behind you. Keep your lower back flat or slightly arched at all times. With your knees just slightly bent, alternate lifting each leg one to six inches from the floor (Figure 2-17). Repeat. This exercise strengthens your rectus abdominis and hip flexors.

Leg raises: Support your back with your elbows. Raise your feet six inches off of the floor (Figure 2-18) and gently lift (Figure 2-19), and then lower them just two inches. The range of motion is from six inches to eight inches. Keep your knees slightly bent at all times. This exercise develops strength in your rectus abdominis and hip flexors.

Scissors: While your elbows support your lower back, extend your legs out in front of you with your knees slightly bent. Cross your right leg over your left (Figure 2-20) then your left leg over your right (Figure 2-21) and repeat. This exercise strengthens your rectus abdominis and hip flexors.

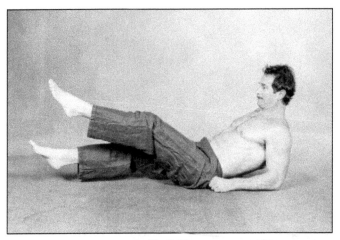

Fig 2-17

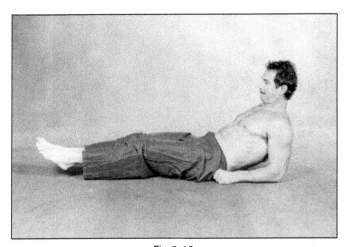

Fig 2-18

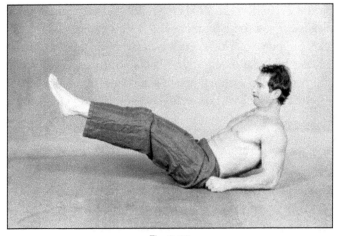

Fig 2-19

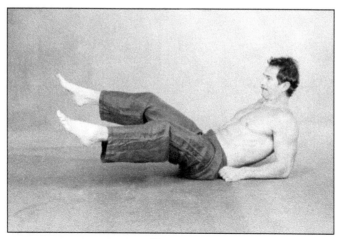

Fig 2-20

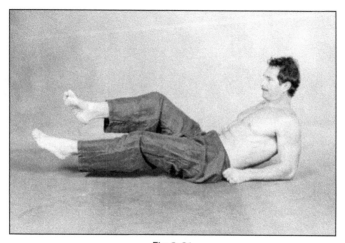

Fig 2-21

Bicycle: While your elbows continue to support your lower back, extend your right leg by straightening your right knee, and retract your left leg by bending your left knee (Figure 2-22). Alternate legs, extending and retracting as if you were riding a bicycle (Figure 2-23). Concentrate on working your rectus abdominis and hip flexors.

Leg extensions: As your elbows support your back, bring both knees to your chest (Figure 2-24) and then extend your legs forward until the knees are slightly bent (Figure 2-25). Repeat. This exercise develops your rectus abdominis and hip flexors.

Elbow to opposite knee: While you lie on your back with your knees bent, interlock your fingers behind your head. Raise your right elbow to your left knee without pulling on your neck with your hands (Figure 2-26). You should feel the tension in the upper right quadrant of your abdomen. Repeat with your left elbow reaching towards your right knee. This exercise strengthens your obliques.

Pulsing: With your knees bent, lift your head and shoulders three inches off the floor (Figure 2-27). Contract the abdominal muscles, without using your neck and back. Repeat.

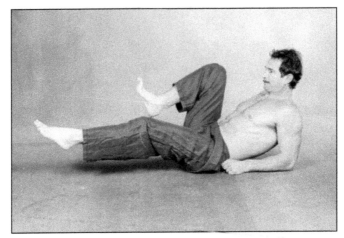

Fig 2-22

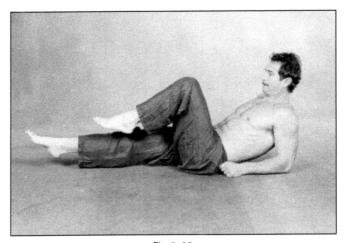

Fig 2-23

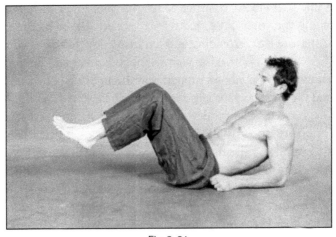

Fig 2-24

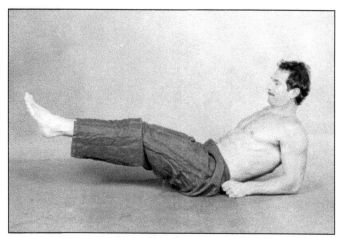

Fig 2-25

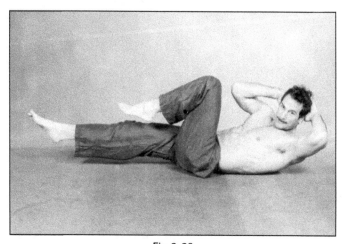

Fig 2-26

Feet up: Raise your feet straight up and keep your knees slightly bent (Figure 2-28). Interlock your fingers behind your head and contract your abdominals by bringing your elbows up toward your knees without pulling with your hands (Figure 2-29). Contract and then release. Repeat.

Feet out: Allow your legs to stretch out to the sides with your knees slightly bent (Figure 2-30). Extend your arms out to the front as you lift your head and shoulders three inches off the floor (Figure 2-31). Use your abdominals to pull your hands between your legs. Repeat.

Opposite Extend: Lie on your back with your knees up. Interlock your fingers behind your head (Figure 2-32) . Contract your abdominals in order to pull your right elbow up to your left knee as you simultaneously extend your right leg (Figure 2-33). Bring your left elbow to your right knee and extend your left leg. Repeat.

Right leg up: While on your back, prop your right foot up on your left knee. Interlock your fingers behind your head (Figure 2-34). Contract your obliques as you

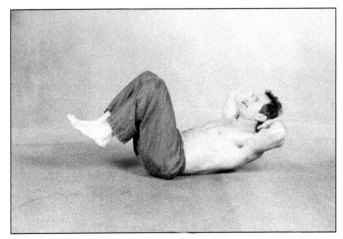

Fig 2-27

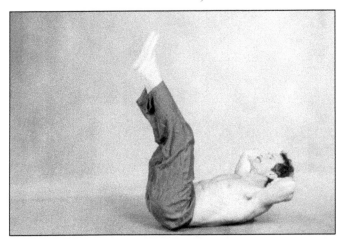

Fig 2-28

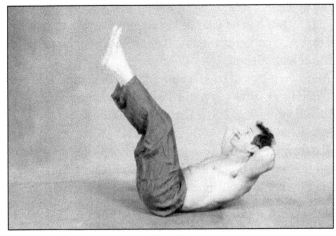

Fig 2-29

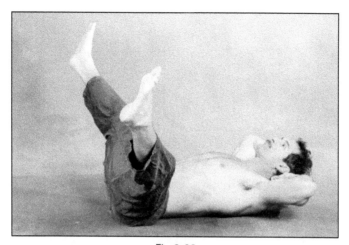

Fig 2-30

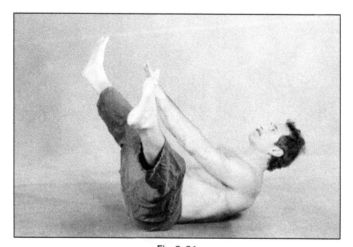

Fig 2-31

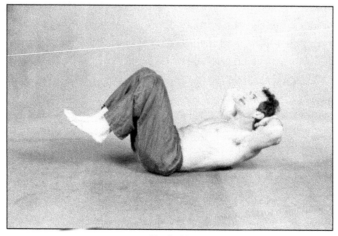

Fig 2-32

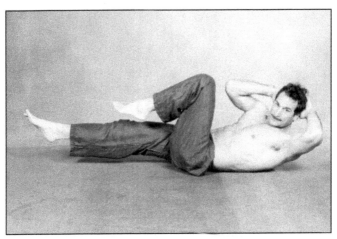

Fig 2-33

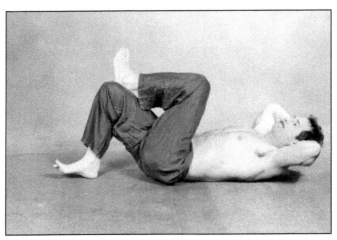

Fig 2-34

raise your left elbow toward your right knee (Figure 2-35). Release the tension, then repeat. Without changing the position of your legs, raise your right elbow towards your right knee (Figure 2-36). Repeat. Then switch the position of your legs, so your left foot is propped on your right knee. Repeat the sequence.

Waist Exercises

Perform your waist exercises along with your abdominal routine. Perform all the waist exercises while lying on the right side of your body. Maintain perfect posture and proper form. Keep your spine in alignment. When you have completed all the exercises on your right side, switch to your left side and repeat each sequence. Perform ten repetitions of each exercise. Add two repetitions each week until you can do twenty.

Slowly down: Lie on your side with your feet together and your knees straight (Figure 2-37). Raise both legs three feet to the side (Figure 2-38) and bring them down slowly. This exercise works the muscles in your waist and hip (obliques and abductors).

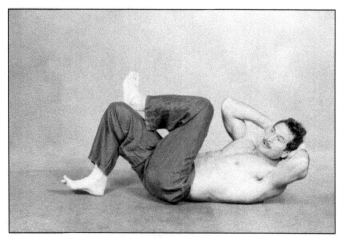

Fig 2-35

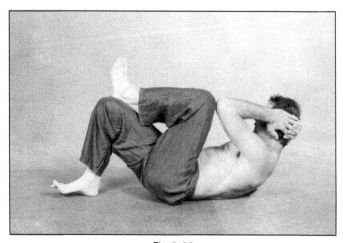

Fig 2-36

Top leg over the other: While lying on your side, cross your top leg over your bottom leg (Figure 2-39). Attempt to lift the lower leg three inches from the floor (Figure 2-40). Focus your attention on working the muscles in your inner thigh (abducters).

Flex extend: Maintain exactly the same position as you move the top leg over the other, and continue to hold the lower leg three inches off the floor (Figure 2-41). Then flex and extend your ankle as you continue to maintain constant tension in your waist and inner thigh (Figure 2-42).

Top leg up, back, and forward: Remain on your side and lift your top leg up one foot from the floor with your toes pointed down (Figure 2-43). Contract your waist as you lightly pulse your leg one inch up and down (Figure 2-44). Then bring your foot back, changing the angle of your leg forty-five degrees (Figure 2-45). Continue to pulse it focusing the workload on your waist and lower back area. Next, bring your leg up to a forty-five degree angle forward (Figure 2-46). Continue the small pulsing action to strengthen your obliques and abductors.

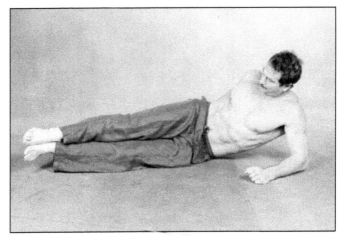

Fig 2-37

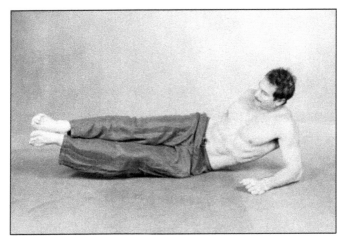

Fig 2-38

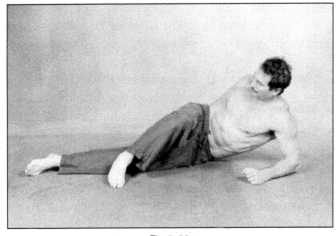

Fig 2-39

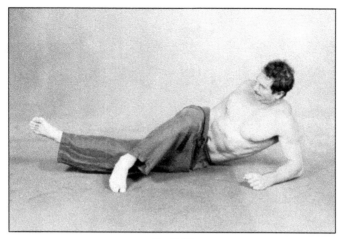

Fig 2-40

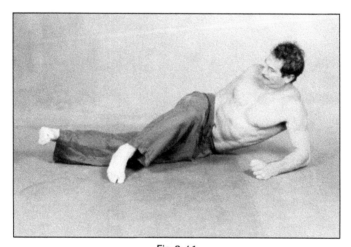

Fig 2-41

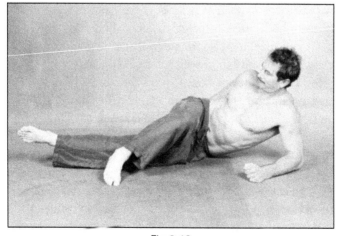

Fig 2-42

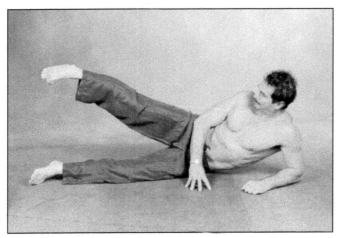

Fig 2-43

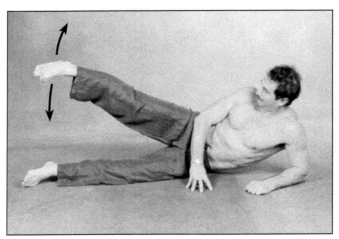

Fig 2-44

Both feet at the same time: The next sequence requires that you hold your legs together and lift them both three inches off the floor (Figure 2-47). Gently lift and lower your legs without touching the ground, pulsing them as they remain together, concentrating the muscular tension in your hip and obliques.

Alternate feet: Lift your top leg one foot off the floor (Figure 2-48). Bring the bottom leg up until it touches the top leg (Figure 2-49). Then lower the bottom leg to the floor (Figure 2-50). Finally, bring the top leg down to the bottom leg as you concentrate on working your adductors and abductors (Figure 2-51). Repeat.

One leg up to the other: Lift your top leg three feet off the floor (Figure 2-52). As you hold your top leg in a static position, bring the bottom leg up until it touches the top leg (Figure 2-53). Let your bottom leg come back down to the floor (Figure 2-54) and repeat. Focus the tension in your obliques, adductors, and abductors.

Elbow to your hip: Bend your knees, keeping your legs together (Figure 2-55). Interlock your fingers behind your neck. Gently lift your top elbow towards your hip, concentrating on the tension in your obliques (Figure 2-56). Repeat.

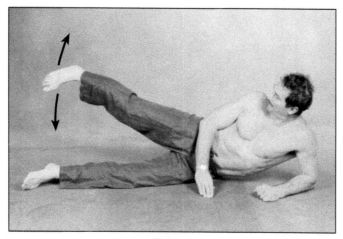

Fig 2-45

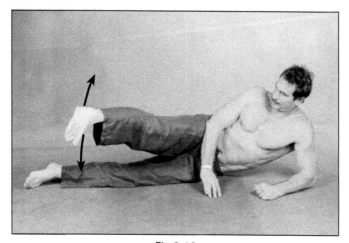

Fig 2-46

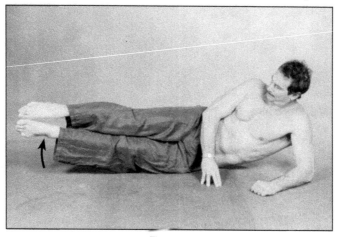

Fig 2-47

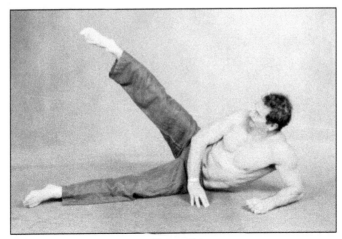

Fig 2-48

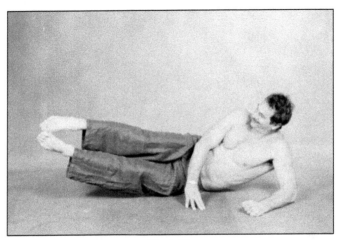

Fig 2-49

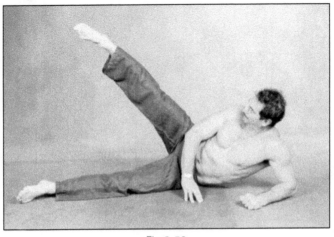

Fig 2-50

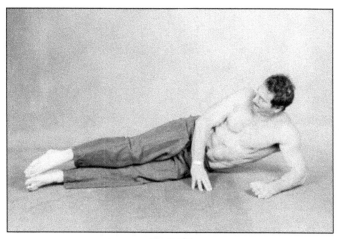

Fig 2-51

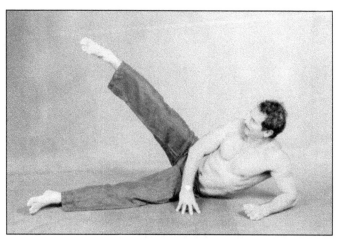

Fig 2-52

Knees up pulse: Allow your elbow and hip to support your weight. Keep your knees together and pulse them up and down two inches (Figure 2-57). Feel the tension in your obliques.

Wrap around pressing up: Lie on your left side with your knees slightly bent. Wrap your right arm across your body so it supports your body weight (Figure 2-58). Extend your right arm up and down as you feel tension in your obliques and triceps (Figure 2-59).

Elbow to knee: Lie on your left side with your fingers lightly interlocked behind your head (Figure 2-60). Raise your upper body one inch from the floor. Bend your right knee and lift it towards your right elbow (Figure 2-61). Feel the tension in the right quadrant of your obliques.

Knee up—extend: Use a stool or hold the wall for balance with your right hand. Lift your left leg up from the floor, keeping your knee bent (Figure 2-62). When you

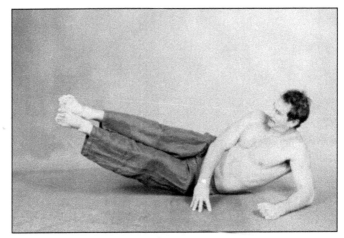

Fig 2-53

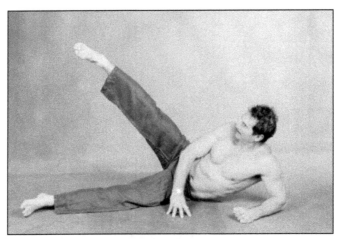

Fig 2-54

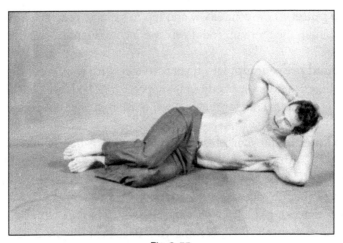

Fig 2-55

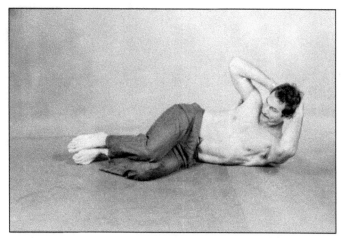

Fig 2-56

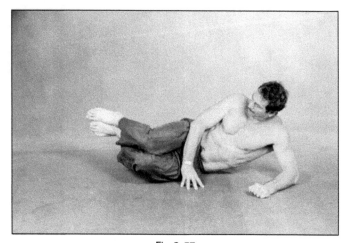

Fig 2-57

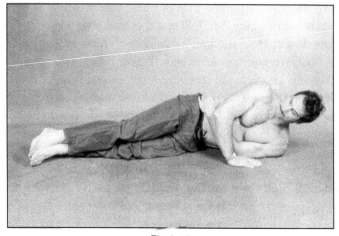

Fig 2-58

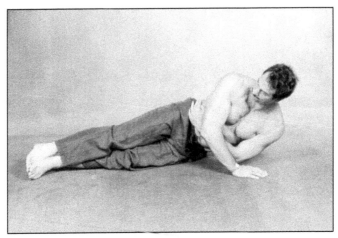

Fig 2-59

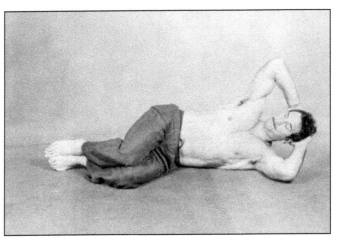

Fig 2-60

raise your knee to the point of tension in your waist, slowly extend your foot until your knee is just slightly bent (Figure 2-63). Flex and extend your leg for ten repetitions.

Toes slightly down: Hold the wall for balance with your right hand. Lift your left leg up from the floor, keeping your knee bent (Figure 2-62). When you raise your knee to the point of tension in your waist and hip, slowly extend your foot, with your toes pointed slightly down (Figure 2-64). Flex and extend your leg for ten repetitions.

Toes all the way down: Hold a chair for balance with your right hand. Lift your left leg up from the floor, keeping your knee bent (Figure 2-62). When you raise your knee to the point of tension in the back of your hip, turn your toes down to the floor and slowly extend your leg (Figure 2-65). Flex and extend your leg for ten repetitions.

Toes down, pull back from the hip: Hold a chair for balance with your right hand. Lift your left leg up from the floor, keeping your knee bent (Figure 2-62). When you raise your knee to the point of tension in the back of your hip, turn your toes down to the floor and slowly extend your leg (Figure 2-66). Keep your leg extended as you pulse your entire leg two inches up and down from the hip (Figure 2-67). Pulse for ten repetitions.

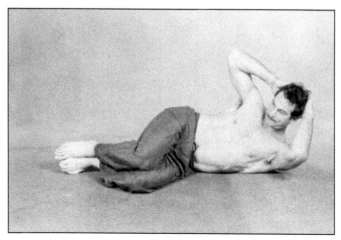

Fig 2-61

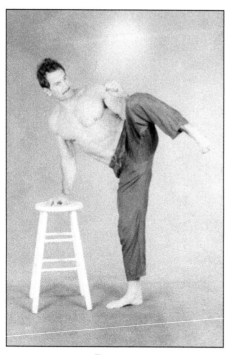

Fig 2-62

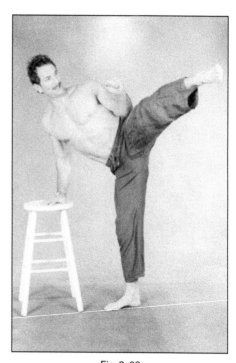

Fig 2-63

Toes sideways, pull up from the waist: Hold a chair for balance with your right hand. Lift your left leg up from the floor, keeping your knee bent (Figure 2-62). When you raise your knee to the point of tension in your waist, extend your leg. Keep your leg extended as you pulse your entire leg two inches up and down from the hip (Figure 2-68). Pulse for ten repetitions.

Circle forward and back: Hold a chair for balance with your right hand. Lift your left leg up from the floor, keeping your knee bent (Figure 2-62). When you raise your knee to the point of tension in your waist, extend your leg. Keep your leg extended and make a small circular movement ten times (Figure 2-69). Then reverse the circle ten times.

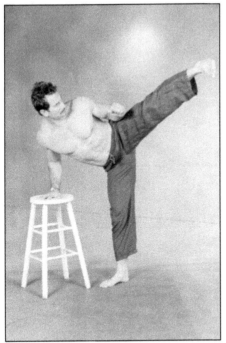

Fig 2-64

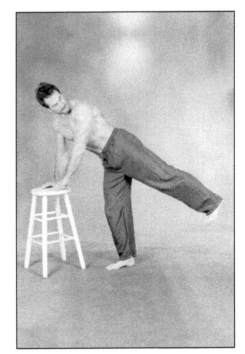

Fig 2-65

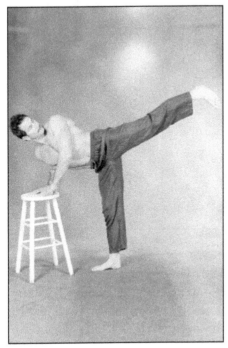

Fig 2-66

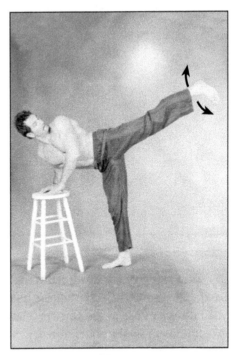

Fig 2-67

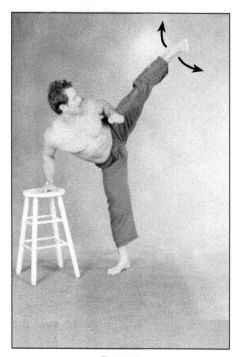

Fig 2-68

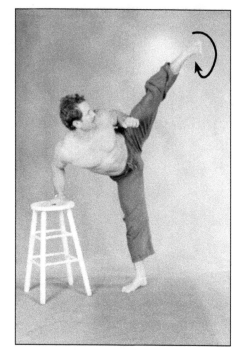

Fig 2-69

Isometric waist and hip toner: Hold a chair for balance with your right hand. Lift your left leg up from the floor, keeping your knee bent (Figure 2-62). When you raise your knee to the point of tension in your waist, extend your leg. Keep your leg extended, with your toes pointed sideways (Figure 2-70). Hold this position for three seconds. Then turn your toes slightly down so you feel the tension in your waist and hip (Figure 2-71). Hold for three seconds. Finally, turn your toes all the way down so you feel the tension in the back of your hip (Figure 2-72). Hold for three seconds.

Knee up—pulse: Hold a chair for balance with your right hand. Lift your left leg up from the floor, keeping your knee bent. When you feel tension in your waist, pulse your knee up and down two inches, for ten repetitions (Figure 2-73).

More About Abdominal Training

You already possess abdominal muscles, without having to do a single sit up or crunch. However, they are probably concealed by a layer of fat. If you are interested in seeing your abs, you must combine abdominal training with aerobic exercise, and a good eating program. Abdominal training firms and strengthens your abs while the aerobic exercise helps to burn off the fat layer that covers them. Punches, kicks, strikes and blocks practiced at a brisk pace is a great way to combine aerobic exercise with your martial arts practice.

In addition, doing abdominal exercises is a warm up before your full workout. Warming up prepares your body for training or competition. Swimmers get ready for their contest with a few easy laps, sprinters run in place, and batters take a few practice

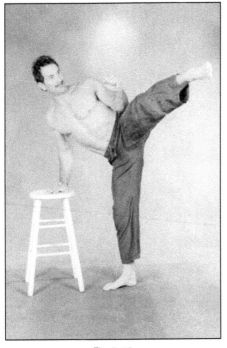

Fig 2-70

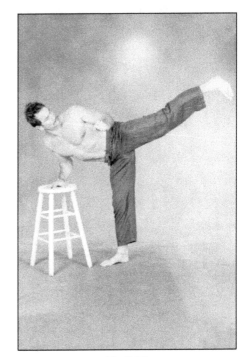

Fig 2-71

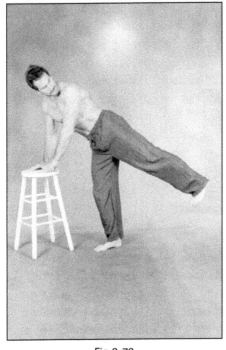

Fig 2-72

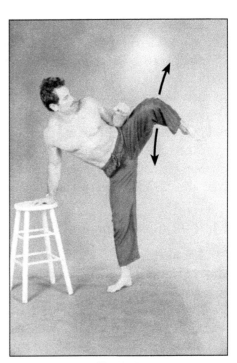

Fig 2-73

swings. Total body exercises such as calisthenics and jumping rope are excellent warm ups. Calisthenics include abdominal training. Abdominal exercises help to raise your overall body temperature, which better prepares your muscles for the workout ahead.

⊃Tips on Abdominal Training

1. You can train abdominals as a warm up before practice.
2. Gradually increase the intensity of your abdominal training until you sweat lightly.
3. Warm up as close to your training as possible so you don't cool down.
4. Warm up a little more in cold weather.
5. Slowly curl up on crunches and reverse crunches, "feel" the movement.
6. Place your hands under your hips to support your back.
7. Don't do too many repetitions. You will not be able to rise from bed the next day.
8. Abdominal training will provide you the confidence to handle body punches.
9. Always maintain a slight arch to your lower back or hold it flat to the floor.

2.2 A Strong Back

Eighty percent of martial artists have, or will have low back pain at some time in their lives. Chronic pain in the lower back may be attributed to weak abdominal muscles, tight hamstrings, poor technique, biomechanical abnormalities, or muscle imbalance. Another cause is the abdominal craze created by "ripped" martial artists on the silver screen. Many unenlightened, would-be action heroes desire a 'six pack' and they purchase all of the fad, fraud infomercial devices to meet that end. Some of these contraptions are biomechanically correct, but others actually trigger low back pain.

If you weigh 150 pounds, there are 100 pounds of intra-disc pressure when you stand, and 140 pounds when you are seated. Straight leg sit-ups place a whopping 210 pounds of pressure on your discs (crunches are responsible for creating 140 pounds of stress). Imagine the torsion stress to your spine when performing ten repetitions of a jump-spinning-hook-kick.

If your job requires you to stand or sit for hours without a break, make an effort to change positions as often as possible. Take frequent strolls to the water fountain. Adjust your chair so your feet are flat on the floor and your knees are bent comfortably. Arm supports reduce disc pressure by fifty percent. When you are required to lift an object off the floor, bend from your knees and hold it close to your body. Consult you physician when necessary.

Signs and symptoms of chronic low back problems include sleeplessness, and pain when standing, sitting, walking, or performing basic martial arts movements. The lumbosacral region including L4, L5, and S1 house the roots to the sciatic nerve (Figure 2-74). Sciatic problems may radiate down either or both legs. Nerve impingement, muscle spasms, spondylolisthesis, and disc problems are just a few of many abnormalities that intensify suffering.

Muscle spasms in your lower back can be comforted with ice. If you don't have ice cubes or an ice pack, you can create an ice pack out of frozen vegetables. Whatever you use, be sure to wrap the pack in a towel or cloth. Treat your lower back muscles (erector spinae) for ten to fifteen minutes several times a day.

Lower Back Strength and Flexibility

A healthy lower back is a result of lower body strength and flexibility, and necessary for a strong torso overall. The following exercises work the lumbar area

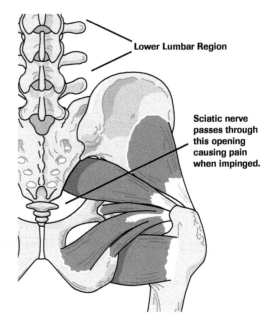

Fig 2-74. Sources of Lower Back Pain

of the back. Progress gradually through this program, paying particular attention to stiffness or pain in the lower back area. Start off slowly, and progress easily.

Flutter kick: Lie on your stomach with your arms out in front. Perform a flutter kick with your feet, as your arms remain off the floor pointing straight ahead (Figure 2-75).

Scissors: While your arms remain out in front, perform a scissors action with your legs, crossing one leg over the other and reversing it (Figure 2-76).

Your upper and lower back can also be improved by doing the "Superman" exercise. The technical name is the prone arm and leg lift. Lie on your stomach. Hold both arms in front of your body, and lift your legs off the ground. Two or three inches is sufficient. Hold for three seconds, relax, and then repeat.

Stretching, which will be discussed in more detail later, may also help alleviate chronic back pain. For quick relief, lie on your side and curl up in a fetal position (Figure 2-77). Flip onto your back and pull one knee to your chest, then the other (Figure 2-78), and then both simultaneously (Figure 2-79). Roll to your stomach with your hands shoulder width apart. Raise up onto your hands and knees while you lift your back into a "mad cat" position (Figure 2-80). Finish up with your favorite thigh (quadriceps), hamstrings (biceps femoris), and hip (gluteal) stretches.

Stretch slowly and continuously while doing these movement. Exhale as you move into each position. Learn to hold your stretch for at least twenty seconds to fully relax the muscles. This will allow for a greater and more comfortable stretch. Slowly stretch to the limits of joint motion, then relax. Soft music in the background is nice. Monitor your joints, muscles, and tendons. Perform an inventory of your back. No pain is gain.

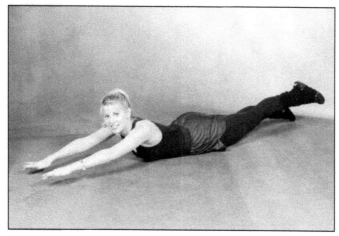

Fig 2-75

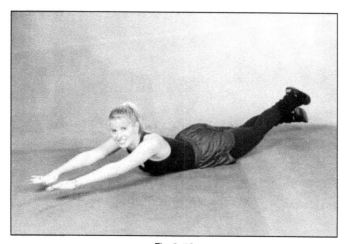

Fig 2-76

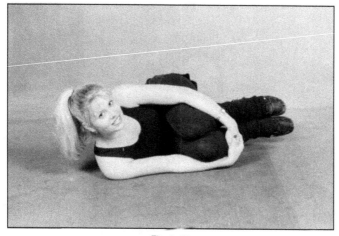

Fig 2-77

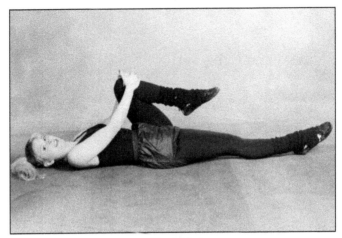

Fig 2-78

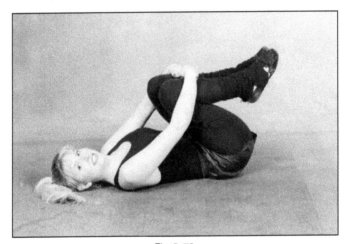

Fig 2-79

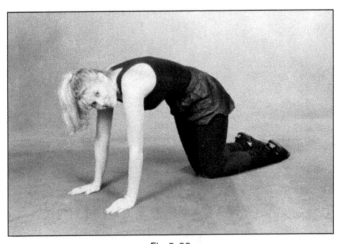

Fig 2-80

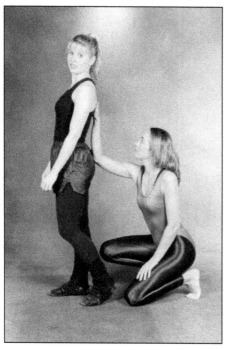

Fig 2-81

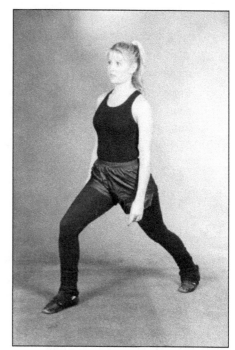

Fig 2-82

The suppleness of your body affects the flexibility of your mind. A theory suggests low back pain begins and ends in your brain. Proponents of this hypothesis suggest that you:

a. Avoid stressful situations.

b. Change the stressful situation so it is no longer a threat.

c. Or change your reaction to the stressful situation.

A restful night is also helpful. But if pain in your lower back affects the quality of your sleep, try sleeping on your side in a fetal position, or try lying on your back and placing pillows under your knees.

Mind/body unity is important in your martial arts training, and good posture reflects both a strong body and healthy spirit. Tune into your lower back. To do this, find your neutral spine by standing with your back to a wall. Slip your hand in the space between your lower back and the wall. This is your neutral spine (Figure 2-81). Feel the difference when you lessen the arch in your lower back.

Besides posture, the next best way to help support your lower back is to strengthen your quadriceps, hamstrings, and gluteals by doing half-squats or lunges (Figure 2-82).

⊃Low Back Health Tips

1. Avoid twisting your waist, especially when carrying a load.

2. Try not to lift both legs simultaneously with your knees locked.

3. Refrain from rapid movements such as twisting, forward flexion, or hyperextension.

4. When ducking an attack, bend from your knees, not your back.

5. Maintain perfect posture during all martial arts techniques.

6. Practice maintaining a slight arch in your lower back while sitting and standing.

7. Remind yourself of perfect posture all day long.

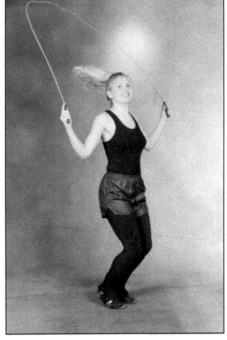

Fig 2-83

2.3 Jumping Rope

After your abdominal workout and lower back exercises, move on to jumping rope. Five minutes of easy skipping is a great way to warm up before your workout. Jump lightly on the balls of your feet with your knees bent to work your calf muscles and take the pressure off your shins and knees. Use your wrists to turn the rope. Hold your hands at your waist about two inches from your body. Jump low. Increase your endurance one minute a week until you can jump for fifteen minutes (Figure 2-83). Jumping rope is also an excellent cardiovascular workout.

⟳Tips on Jumping Rope

1. To measure your rope, stand on the middle of the rope, holding an end in each hand. Each end should reach your armpit.

2. Cotton ropes swing slowly and leather ropes wear out. Plastic is my favorite.

3. Jump rope on wood floors, rubber floors, or rubber tiles.

2.4 Incredible Flexibility

Overseas we never practiced the splits. Instead we used a rope-pulley hanging from the ceiling, with a belt tied to one end. You placed your foot inside the belt loop, tightened it snugly around your ankle, grabbed the other end of the rope and hoisted your leg up as high as possible. You could stretch your hamstring muscles by pulling on the rope with your toes facing straight up, your inner thigh muscles by turning your toes sideways, and your hip muscles by flipping your toes down. When I returned to the United States I was able to perform a full Chinese split on my first attempt.

Flexibility helps you move freely in every direction through a full and normal range of motion (ROM). Flexibility is very individual and is specific to each joint. You may be flexible in your lower body and tight in your upper body, or vice versa. Stretching should be an important part of your overall training program to develop flexibility.

⊃Eight Reasons to Stretch

1. Stretching increases your efficiency of movement. Flexible joints and muscles require less effort to move.
2. Muscle can be stretched 1.6 times resting length before it tearing. Stretching may help prevent injury.
3. Flexibility increases the range of motion around joints. This improves your balance and posture as well as your physical and martial arts skills.
4. Stretching reduces muscle/joint stiffness by increasing the blood and nutrient supply to the joint structures.
5. Stretching reduces the thickness of synovial fluid, allowing for a better nutrient exchange. Stretching may also decelerate degenerative joint changes associated with age and injury.
6. Stretching relieves muscle soreness by increasing the blood and oxygen supply to the area and helps dissipate lactic acid.
7. Stretching encourages relaxation and reduces emotional stress.
8. Stretching is an important part of rehabilitation of injuries.

In general, there are two types of flexibility: static and dynamic. Static flexibility is the ROM around a joint in a motionless position. Holding your legs in a split is an example of static flexibility. Dynamic flexibility describes the ROM around a joint while you're moving. It involves speed. An example of dynamic flexibility is throwing a side kick.

Most of the tension you feel when you stretch is not from your muscle fibers. The connective tissue around the muscle, including your tendons, fascia, and ligaments, provides resistance. Muscle fascia sheaths account for forty-one percent of the resistance, ligaments and joint capsules account for forty-seven percent, tendons ten percent, and skin two percent. One of the goals of your stretching program is to improve the flexibility both of your muscles and the connective tissue.

When connective tissue is lengthened due to force, such as a high side kick, an elastic elongation occurs. But your muscles, fascia, and connective tissue return to their previous resting length when the force is removed, i.e. as your foot returns to the floor. Elastic elongation of your connective tissue is only temporary.

A permanent stretch in your muscle, fascia, and connective tissue is called plastic elongation. This means a new resting length has been attained. Plastic elongation is your key to improved flexibility.

Flexibility exercises require no special equipment other than loose clothing. Stretch after you are thoroughly warmed up. Relax the muscle groups you are working. Exhale as you move into each position. Stretch to a slight level of discomfort, never approaching pain. Do not bounce or jerk. A slow, continuous stretch is desired.

Perform your routine with grace and control. Go as far as it feels comfortable to you. Some days you may be more flexible than others, and at different times of the day. I can always elongate my muscles farther in the afternoon than in the morning. You may find the opposite.

While you are stretching, monitor your joints, muscles, and tendons. Settle into your maximum flexibility pose. Soon your body will adapt and you may go down even further. While you are stretching, perform an inventory on your body to be sure all parts are in perfect working order. Enjoy your routine. The suppleness of your body will affect the flexibility of your mind.

Be sure to stretch after you warm up. Stretching is also an important element for your cool down. After martial arts training, your legs and lower back muscles tighten. Ignoring this stiffness makes things worse, especially if you go from the training hall to the couch. Muscles may tense up even more, causing pain. Stretching after your work-out helps enhance flexibility because warm muscles are inclined to stretch more than usual. Stretching before and after your workout will keep you fit.

The following section presents a modified version of three different types of stretching: Active Isolated (AI) stretching, Proprioceptive Neuromuscular Facilitation (PNF), and static stretching. I recommend combining these three types to get the best results. To perform many martial arts techniques such as high kicks, you require static flexibility to extend your leg. You also need the strength of the supporting muscles to thrust the leg high into the air. Thus, a combination of AI, PNF, and static stretching can help you to optimize your flexibility.

Active Isolated (AI) stretching

When you contract a muscle, its antagonist, or opposing muscle, relaxes. For example if you contract your thigh, your hamstring automatically relaxes. This is called reciprocal inhibition. Active Isolated (AI) stretching is based in this principle.

To perform AI stretching, first decide on the muscle you want to stretch. Then contract the opposing muscle. This automatically allows the muscle you are stretching to relax. Then stretch to the point of light tension. Hold for two seconds. Perform eight to ten repetitions of each stretch. Since the stretch is held for no longer than two seconds, it avoids the "stretch reflex," which would typically cause a contraction in the muscle you are trying to stretch.

The stretch reflex is your body's defense mechanism against over-stretching. Deep in your muscle tissue are muscle spindles. They run parallel to your muscle fibers. They stretch along with your muscle fibers and protect your muscles and tendons. Whenever they sense an excessive stretch, the spindles cause your muscle to reflexively contract. A quick, violent stretch to your muscle, results in a quick, violent contraction. However, as mentioned above, doing AI stretching for only two seconds avoids this stretch reflex.

AI Single Adductor Stretch: Your supporting foot remains flat while you extend your other leg to the side. Flex the quadriceps of your extended leg. Hold for two seconds and then stretch until you feel tension in the inner thigh of your extended leg (Figure 2-84). Hold the stretch for two seconds. Repeat with the other leg.

AI Double Adductor Stretch: Spread your legs out as far as possible supporting your weight from your knees. Flex your quadriceps for two seconds. Let your body weight push you down until you feel tension in your inner thighs (Figure 2-85). Hold at tension for two seconds.

AI Biceps Femoris Stretch: Perform the straddle split. Point your toes up at the ceiling. Flex your quadriceps for three seconds (Figure 2-86). Slowly bring your chest toward the floor while maintaining a neutral spine (Figure 2-87). When you feel tension, hold for two seconds.

AI Chest to Knee: Sit with one leg forward and the other curled inward in a 'figure 4' position. Flex the quadriceps on your front leg and hold for two seconds. Pull your chest toward your knee, and your forehead toward your shin maintaining a neutral spine (Figure 2-88). When you feel tension, hold for two seconds. Repeat with the other leg.

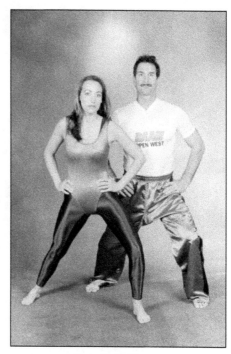

Fig 2-84

AI Chest to Toes: Sit with your back flat and the bottoms of your feet together. Pull your feet in as close to your groin as possible. Flex your quadriceps for two seconds and then grab your toes. Slowly bring your chest toward your toes (Figure 2-89). Hold for two seconds.

AI Butterfly: From the forehead to toes position, flex your quadriceps for two seconds and grab your ankles and push your knees toward the floor with your elbows (Figure 2-90). Hold for two seconds.

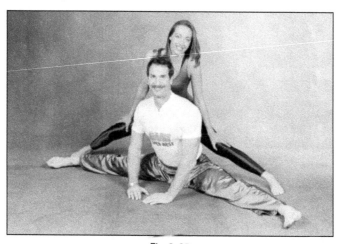

Fig 2-85

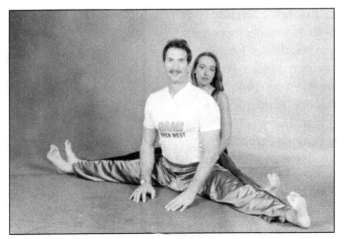

Fig 2-86

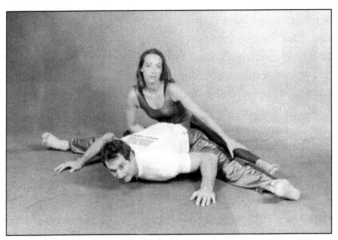

Fig 2-87

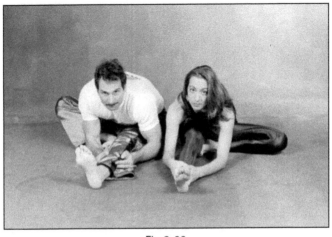

Fig 2-88

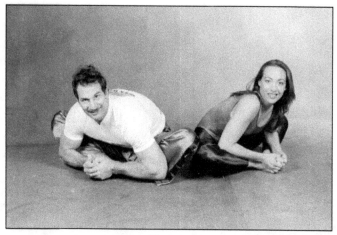

Fig 2-89

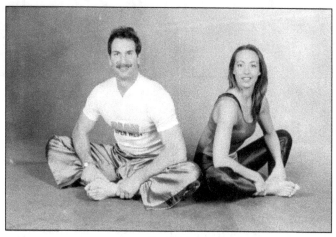

Fig 2-90

AI Quadriceps Stretch: Stand with your left side next to a wall and grab the top of your right foot. Flex the muscles in your right hamstring and hold for two seconds. Then relax and stretch your right quadriceps (thigh) until you feel tension (Figure 2-91). Hold for two seconds. Switch legs and repeat the exercise.

Proprioceptive Neuromuscular Facilitation (PNF)

Proprioceptive neuromuscular facilitation (PNF) is a type of stretching that will provide mega-results. Your partner pulls you slowly into a perfect stretch. When you feel tension, you push against your partner for three seconds, then you relax and allow your partner to pull just a tad more. A partner helps you achieve a greater stretch than you dreamed possible. When working with your partner, move slowly into position. Stretch to the point of tension (not pain), contract the muscle you are stretching, and then relax. It is important that your partner moves slowly through the stretch, contract, relax progression.

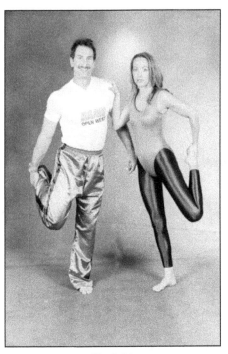

Fig 2-91

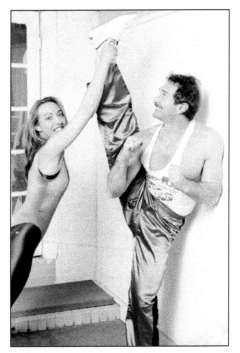

Fig 2-92

PNF Gluteus, Hamstring Wall Stretch: Stand with your back and heels flat against a wall with both knees slightly bent. Let your partner grab your right ankle and slowly lift it until you feel tension (Figure 2-92). When you feel tension, tell your partner to stop. Pull from your right hamstring and press the back of your heel toward the floor while your partner resists for three seconds. Relax and repeat with your left leg.

PNF Gracilis, Adductor Magnus, Longus and Brevis Wall Stretch: Stand facing sideways to the wall with both knees slightly bent. Let your partner grab your right ankle and slowly lift it until you feel tension. Be sure your toes point sideways through the duration of the stretch (Figure 2-93). When you feel tension, tell your partner to stop. Pull from your right inner thigh back toward the floor while your partner resists for three seconds. Relax and repeat with your left leg.

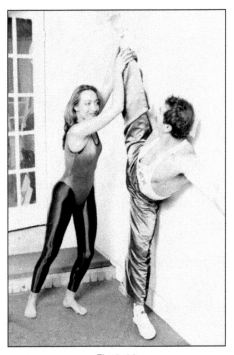

Fig 2-93

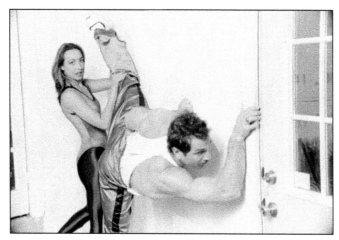

Fig 2-94

PNF Hip Flexor, Rectus Femoris, Wall Stretch: Stand facing the wall with both knees slightly bent. Place your hands comfortably on the wall for balance. Let your partner grab your right ankle and slowly lift it until you feel tension. Be sure the toes on your right foot point down (Figure 2-94). When you feel tension tell your partner to stop. Pull from your hip toward the floor while your partner resists for three seconds. Relax and repeat with your left leg.

Static Stretching

Static Stretching may be the type you are most familiar with. These stretches can be performed both solo and with a partner. Be sure to warm up before doing these stretches.

Achilles Tendon and Calf Stretch:

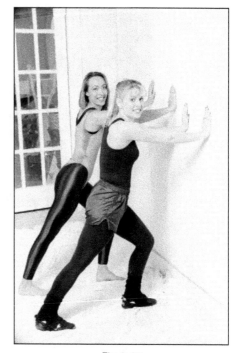

Fig 2-95

Place the palms of both hands on the wall. Extend your right leg back with your knee straight. Your left knee should be out in front and bent. Place eighty percent of your weight on your left leg until you feel a stretch in the calf muscle of your right leg (Figure 2-95). Hold for fifteen seconds, then relax. Repeat with your left leg.

Lower Back Stretch: Lie on your back and attempt to bring your knees slowly to your chest. Then lower your chin to your chest and hold for fifteen seconds (Figure 2-96).

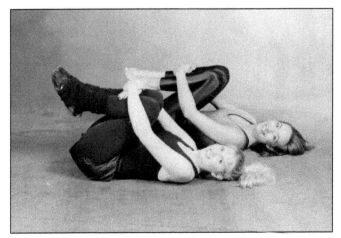

Fig 2-96

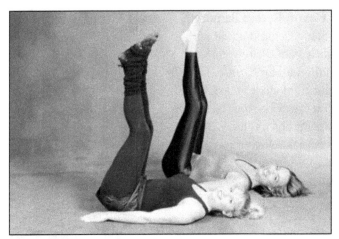

Fig 2-97

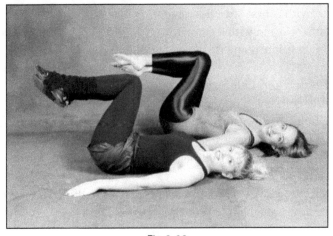

Fig 2-98

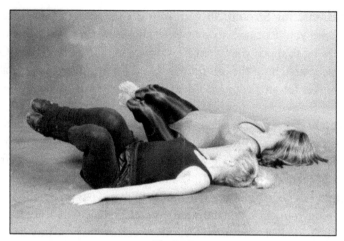

Fig 2-99

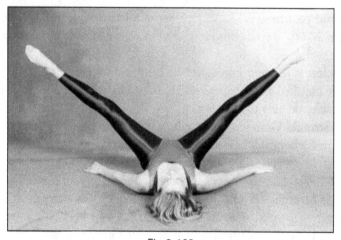

Fig 2-100

Hip Stretch, Waist Toner: Lie flat on your back with your arms extended to the sides. Raise your feet up toward the ceiling with your knees straight. Slowly lower both legs to your right as your eyes look to the left (Figure 2-97). Then, as you bring your legs back up and to the left, simultaneously turn your head so you are looking to your right. Keep constant tension in your hips and waist as you feel the stretch. Repeat back and forth.

Finally, bring both knees up to your chest. As you slowly lower them to your right side, turn your head so you are looking to your left (Figure 2-98). Repeat in the opposite direction (Figure 2-99).

Ultimate Inner Thigh Stretch: Lie on your back with your hips against the wall. Place your hips as close to the wall as possible. Let your legs open and slowly climb down the wall an inch at a time until you feel tension in your inner thighs (Figure 2-100). At the point of tension, make sure your lower back is flat against the floor. Hold for thirty seconds.

Calf and Hamstring Stretch: Sit with your left leg straight forward and your right leg bent with your foot next to your inner thigh. Reach toward the toes of your left foot, attempting to touch your chest to your left knee (Figure 2-101). Grab your toes and pull back, stretching the calf muscle. Hold for fifteen seconds. Grab your ankle and bring your chest towards your left knee (Figure 2-102). Hold for fifteen seconds and release.

Waist Stretch: Bring your inside foot (right foot) across your knee and continue to twist your waist in that same direction (Figure 2-103). Hold for fifteen seconds. Next, rotate in the opposite direction while your foot remains in position. Twist from the waist until you feel tension (Figure 2-104). Hold for fifteen seconds.

Hip Stretch: Lift your right foot onto your thigh so your ankle rests on your left thigh. Slowly bring your chest down toward your ankle until you feel tension in your hip (Figure 2-105). Hold that position for fifteen seconds. Repeat this entire sequence with the other leg.

Alternate Hip Stretch: Cross your left leg in front of your right. Let your chest fall slowly toward your feet. When you feel tension in your left hip, hold for fifteen seconds (Figure 2-106). Repeat this exercise with your right leg in front for fifteen seconds.

Waist Circles: With your knees slightly bent and your hands on your hips, circle your torso three hundred sixty degrees slowly to the right (Figure 2-107). Then circle three hundred sixty degrees to your left.

Shoulder Stretch: Grab your right elbow with your left hand behind your head and pull the arm back until you feel tension (Figure 2-108); hold for fifteen seconds, then relax. Next, bring your right arm across your body and pull gently with your left hand (Figure 2-109). Hold for fifteen seconds. Repeat with your opposite arm.

Quadriceps Stretch: Lie on your left side, with your left arm out in front of you for balance. Bend your right leg at the knee, bringing your heel back towards the back of your right thigh. Grasp your right foot with your right hand and gently push your heel towards your right thigh until you feel tension in your quadriceps (Figure 2-110). Hold for fifteen seconds, then switch sides and repeat the exercise.

Back-to-Back Stretch: Sit back to back with your partner. Extend your legs in a straddle position as your partner presses his or her back to yours and applies slow pressure to your lower back. As he or she pushes gently on your back, allow your chest to move slowly toward the floor in front of you. When you feel tension, hold for fifteen seconds (Figure 2-111). Repeat this sequence with your legs one foot apart. Hold for fifteen seconds until you feel tension.

Next, perform the same back-to-back stretch routine with your knees together. As your partner presses his or her back to yours, slowly attempt to let your chest drop down toward your knees. When you feel tension in your hamstrings, hold for fifteen seconds (Figure 2-112). Finally, bring the soles of your feet together. As your partner applies pressure to your lower back, he or she simultaneously pushes on your knees with equal pressure (Figure 2-113). As you feel tension on your inner thighs and hips, hold for fifteen seconds.

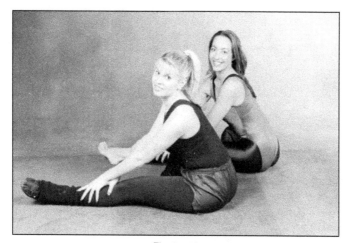

Fig 2-101

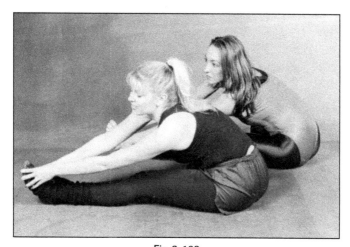

Fig 2-102

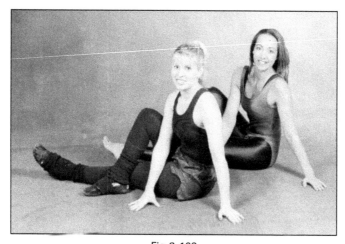

Fig 2-103

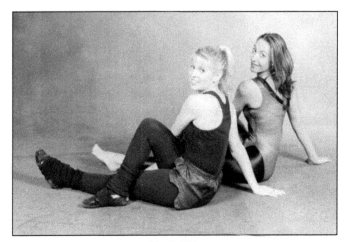

Fig 2-104

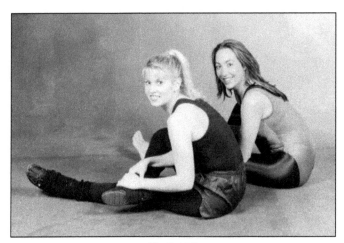

Fig 2-105

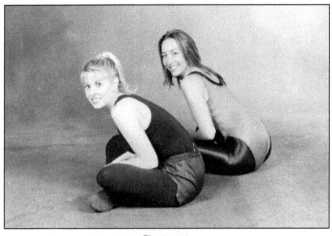

Fig 2-106

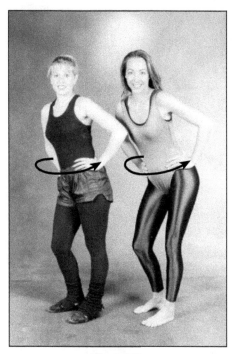

Fig 2-107

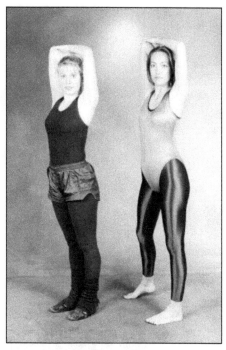

Fig 2-108

Neck Stretch: Bring your chin straight down to your chest (Figure 2-114). Hold for fifteen seconds. Then allow your chin to lift up toward the ceiling as you lift your shoulders (Figure 2-115). When you feel tension, hold for fifteen seconds. Pull your left ear toward your left shoulder (Figure 2-116). Hold at the point of tension for fifteen seconds. Finally, let your right ear come toward your right shoulder until you feel tension. Hold for fifteen seconds.

Wall Stretches

Achilles tendon stretch: Face the wall with your hands shoulder width apart and your right leg back. Slowly transfer your weight to your left leg (Figure 2-117). Feel a stretch in your right achilles tendon. Hold for fifteen seconds. Repeat with your other leg.

Hip and waist stretch: Face sideways to the wall and lean your hip slowly toward

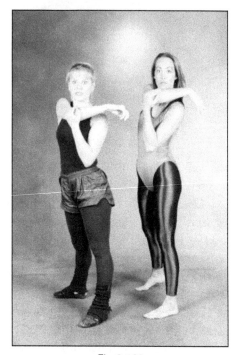

Fig 2-109

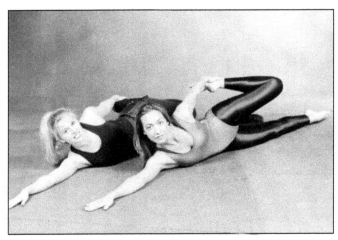

Fig 2-110

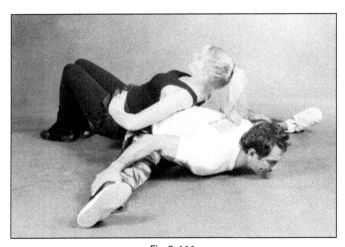

Fig 2-111

the wall (Figure 2-118). When you feel tension, hold for fifteen seconds. Switch sides and repeat.

Chest stretch: Place the palm of your left hand on the wall with your arm extended. Slowly turn to your right until you feel a stretch in your left pectoral muscle (Figure 2-119). Hold for fifteen seconds. Repeat with your right hand.

Inner thigh stretch: Hold onto the wall with your left hand to keep your balance. With your right hand, grab your right knee and lift it up until you feel tension (Figure 2-120). Hold for fifteen seconds.

Back leg lift: Place both hands on the wall. Look over your left shoulder and extend your left leg back (Figure 2-121). Slowly, and with control, lift your extended left leg back and forth five times. Repeat with your right leg.

Side leg lift: Place your left hand on the wall for balance. Look over your right shoulder and extend your right leg out to the side; lift your leg up and down for five repetitions (Figure 2-122). Repeat with your left leg.

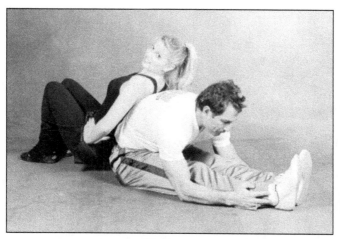

Fig 2-112

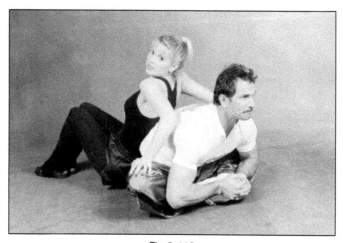

Fig 2-113

Back stretch: Place your palms out in front of you on the floor. Push up slowly from your waist until your arms are extended (Figure 2-123). When your feel a stretch in the abdominals and lower back, hold for fifteen seconds, then relax. If you have lower back problems, raise to your elbows only.

⊃Tips on Stretching

1. Warm up before you stretch.
2. Flex the opposing muscle seconds before you stretch.
3. A slow, continuous stretch is desired.
4. Slowly stretch until you feel tension in your muscle. Then relax. Go for comfort. Settle into your pose.
5. Exhale as you move into each position.
6. Learn to hold your static stretch at least fifteen seconds in order to fully relax

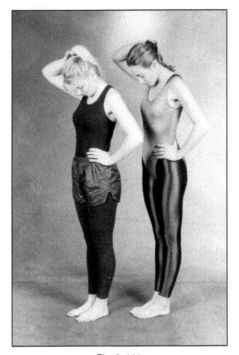

Fig 2-114

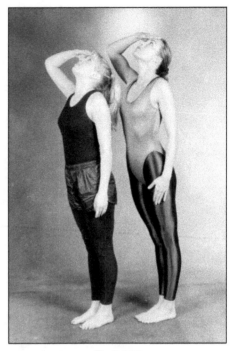

Fig 2-115

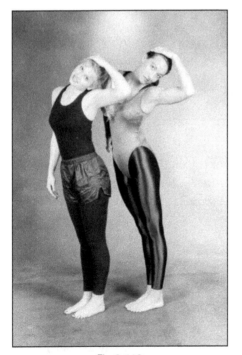

Fig 2-116

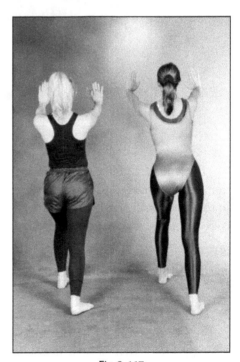

Fig 2-117

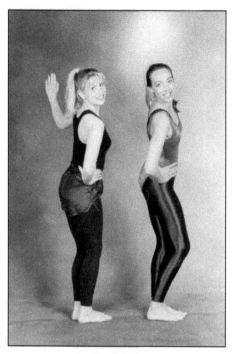

Fig 2-118

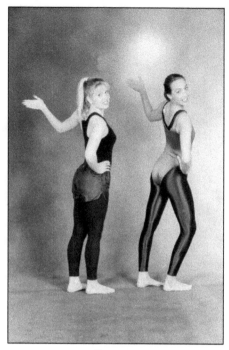

Fig 2-119

the muscle. Add two seconds a week until you work up to thirty seconds for each stretch.

7. Stretch to a slight level of discomfort—not pain.

8. Give your body time to adapt.

9. Practice slow, high kicks to strengthen stabilizer muscles.

2.5 Isometric Stances

One morning I opened the sliding door to the martial arts school and no one was there. I walked up the stairs to the hotel, looked into a tiny room and was surprised to see my seventy-five year old master curled up in a ball, napping. There was little else in the room except his tatami mat. He looked so small and frail. He stood only four feet eleven inches, but on the training floor he was in control. I was a foot taller than he, but in a

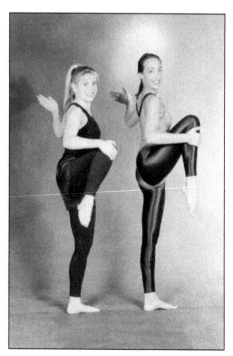

Fig 2-120

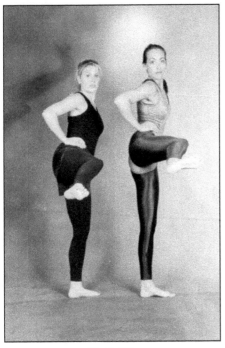

Fig 2-121

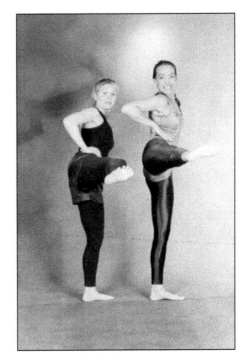

Fig 2-122

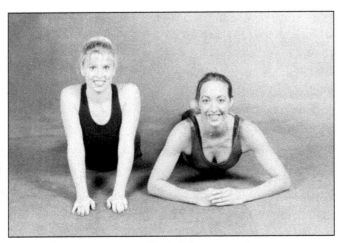

Fig 2-123

fight I would bet on him. My master was the most powerful man pound for pound I've ever seen.

The power in your technique is generated from your legs and hips. When you throw, strike or kick, a dominant but equal force is generated in both directions. To hit through a target, you must shift your weight and relax into a rock-solid stance. Training isometric stances will give you a strong base of support to do so. Hold each stance for three seconds and proceed to the next without rest.

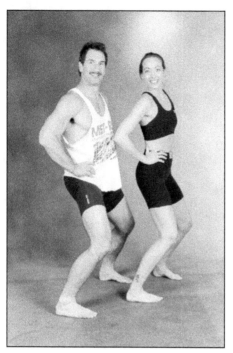

Fig 2-124

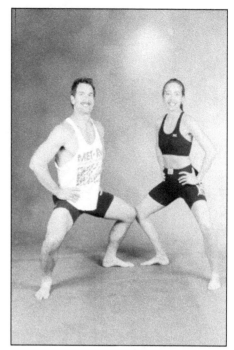

Fig 2-125

Horse riding stance: Stand with your feet shoulder width apart, toes pointed straight ahead, knees slightly bowed, as if you were riding a horse (Figure 2-124). Bend your knees so a string dropped from each knee would hit your big toe. Squeeze the cheeks of your buttocks together and contract your abdominals. Keep your back straight.

Square stance: Change your feet from the horse stance to a left foot forward square stance. To do this, slide your right foot back and to the side so it is perpendicular to your left foot (Figure 2-125). Trace a perfect square with your feet. Bend both knees and keep your back straight.

Square stance heels off: (Same as square stance except the heels are off of the floor.) This exercise is good muscular endurance training for your upper and lower legs. It is outstanding for the calves (Figure 2-126).

Lean front stance: Pivot from your square stance to a right leg-lean front stance. Transfer your weight to your right leg as you lean sideways (Figure 2-127). Switch legs and repeat.

Front stance balance: Change your square stance to a front stance by placing your left leg back and your right leg forward. Bend your right knee over your toe and lift your left leg off the floor. Continue to balance your left leg in the air with your weight over the right knee (Figure 2-128). Hold your back leg straight. Switch legs and repeat.

Cat stance: Switch your front stance to a cat stance by shifting seventy percent of your weight to your back leg. Balance the rest of your weight on the ball of your front foot (Figure 2-129). Switch legs and repeat.

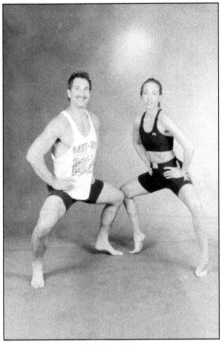

Fig 2-126

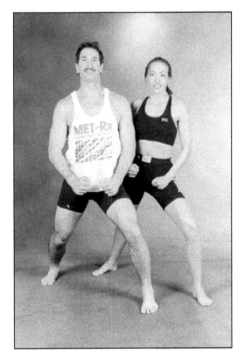

Fig 2-127

Front stance knee down: Assume a front stance with your left leg forward. Bend your right knee so that it comes within one inch of the floor (Figure 2-130). Switch legs and repeat.

Hourglass stance: Stand in a horse stance with your feet shoulder width apart and then turn your toes inward (Figure 2-131).

Back stance: From your hourglass stance, pivot on your heels so your toes are pointing out (Figure 2-132).

Cross walk: From your back stance, cross a leg behind the other and bend both knees (Figure 2-133). Your knees are bent throughout the exercise. Your head and shoulders remain parallel as you travel back and forth across the floor.

Toe-balance, heels out: Place your feet close together with your heels spread apart. Lift your heels off the floor as you rise up on the balls of your feet (Figure 2-134).

Toe-balance, heels in: Touch your heels together as you rise on the balls of your feet (Figure 2-135).

⊃Tips on Stances

1. Practice stances often until you can do them without analysis.
2. Maintain perfect posture: Hold your eyes up, lower back slightly arched, shoulders parallel, stomach in, buttocks tucked under, and your knees soft.
3. At first, hold each stance for three seconds. Add two seconds each week until you can maintain them for thirty seconds.
4. Look straight ahead and focus on your breathing.

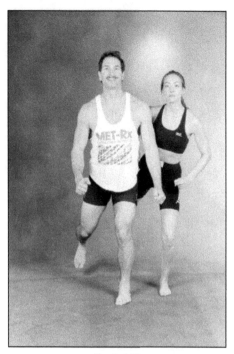

Fig 2-128

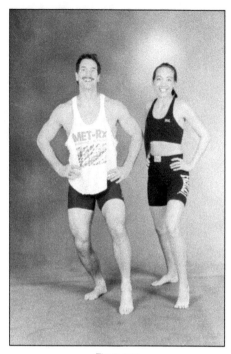

Fig 2-129

5. Perform stance training at least three days per week.

6. Work out in a comfortable room where you won't be interrupted.

2.6 Plyometrics for Explosive Power

In my first martial arts tournament I won my opening two fights by getting bopped on the nose. (Punching to the face is a foul in some martial arts tournaments, resulting in disqualification). I was a semi-finalist but my face looked like I had been hit by a truck. That is the last thing I remember. In the semi-final bout I attempted a rear leg round-house kick. My opponent jumped high into the air and whirled around scoring with a perfect flying spinning hook kick to my neck. Witnesses say they had never seen a kick like

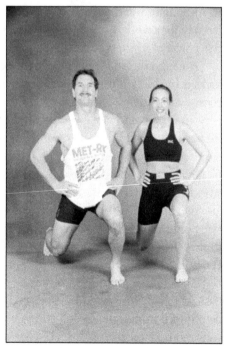

Fig 2-130

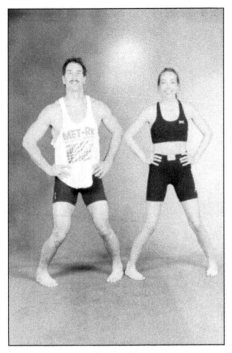

Fig 2-131

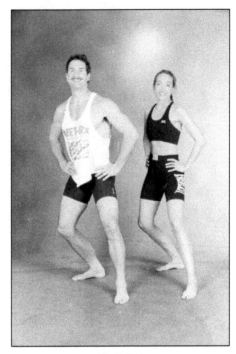

Fig 2-132

it. Although I could not talk or breathe comfortably for a week, I was awed by the deceptive power of my opponent's technique.

A method to add some height to your kicks is by doing plyometrics. Plyometrics consist of a variety of drills that train your nervous system and metabolic pathways to increase your strength and power. Plyometrics requires you to accelerate through a complete range of motion and then relax into a full stretch. Plyometric training will build your fast-twitch muscle fibers, which are the explosive power muscles in your body, as compared to slow-twitch muscle fibers, which are for endurance.

The number of muscle fibers and type (fast twitch or slow twitch) in your body was determined during the second trimester of your mother's pregnancy. Each of your muscle fibers is composed of seventy-five percent water, twenty percent protein, and five percent phosphates, calcium, magnesium, sodium, potassium, chloride, fats, carbohydrates, and

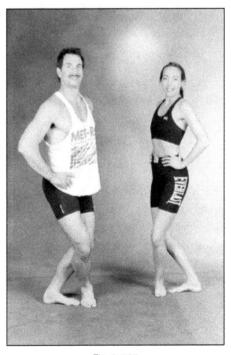

Fig 2-133

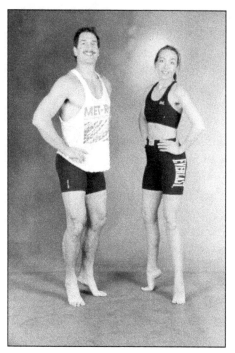

Fig 2-134

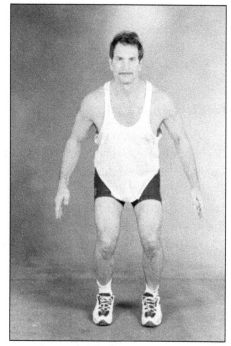

Fig 2-135

amino acids. You have 430 voluntary muscles which represents forty to fifty percent of your body weight. Skeletal muscle is the largest single tissue in your body. Plyometrics pre-stretches your fast-twitch fibers followed by a full-range explosive muscular contraction. Fast twitch and slow twitch are discussed in greater detail in chapter five, in the section on resistance training.

Plyometric Exercises:

Plyometric training is an excellent method for improving your power. You can use plyometrics to allow you to train at a larger percentage of your aerobic capacity so your workouts will feel easier. Plyometrics will also add some snap to your kicks.

Before beginning plyometric training be sure to warm up and stretch. Take it easy on your first few sets and repetitions of plyometrics. Spend at least thirty seconds resting between sets but perform each repetition consecutively. After a month of plyometrics, spend less time between sets and increase to two sets of twenty repetitions.

1. Skip with an exaggerated knee-lift and longer than usual stride, up a hill. Jog down. Do it ten times.
2. Sprint up a hill raising your knees high, and jog down. Do it ten times.
3. Perform ten consecutive standing broad jumps.
4. Perform ten consecutive very short hops.
5. Jump up and down ten times as quickly as you can keeping your feet as close to the ground as possible.

6. Improve leg power and kicking strength by finding a bench about two feet high and stand on it with both knees slightly bent. Jump softly off the end of the bench into a squat stretch. At the bottom of the stretch position immediately bound back onto the bench. Perform ten repetitions.

More Plyometrics

Bounding: Jump up. Land on the balls of your feet and bend your knees to ninety degrees and roll to your heels (Figure 2-136). Then roll to the balls of your feet and jump up nine more times. Do not rest between jumps.

Dive Jumps: Take a three-step running start and bound off both feet, throwing your arms in the air (like Superman jumping out a window) (Figure 2-137). After landing (on your feet, not your face), take three steps back and continue nine more times.

Clap Your Feet: Begin with your feet a little less than shoulder width apart (Figure 2-138). Jump up and touch your feet together (penguin style) (Figure 2-139), then land solidly in your original position. Do ten repetitions.

Evade the Sweep: Jump and bring your heels to your hips (Figure 2-140). Imagine you are evading your opponent's sweep. Be mindful of your knees. Do ten repetitions.

Breakfall: From a standing position (Figure 2-141), roll onto your back and slap the floor with the palms of your hands (Figure 2-142). Rise to a standing position as quickly as you can without using your arms. Do ten repetitions.

Flying Double Front Kick: Jump up and throw front kicks simultaneously. Thrust your fists between your legs on each jump. Do ten repetitions.

Lunge jumps: Begin in a forward lunge position, similar to the front stance in the stance pulse program (Figure 2-143). Jump up and switch stances in the air so each foot replaces the other (Figure 2-144). Take no rest between jumps.

Fingers touch: Touch your fingers to the floor (Figure 2-145) and bound up as high as you can (Figure 2-146). Monitor your knees and back. Do ten repetitions.

⤴Tips on Plyometrics

1. The only requirement is a cushioned floor or grass.
2. When you begin plyometric training, jump no more than two inches high.
3. Add one inch a week until you are jumping at your maximum height.
4. If you are in great shape, repeat the circuit.
5. After a month of training, you may increase to three sets of twenty repetitions.
6. Because of joint stress, perform plyometrics a maximum of once a week.
7. Monitor your knees and ankles and always warm up and stretch before plyometrics.
8. Pre-stretch movements in martial arts (e.g. cocking your technique) creates more power in your strike or kick.

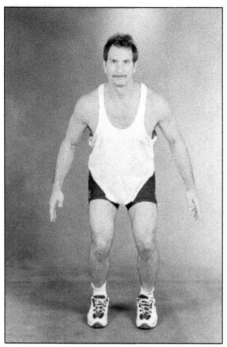

Fig 2-136

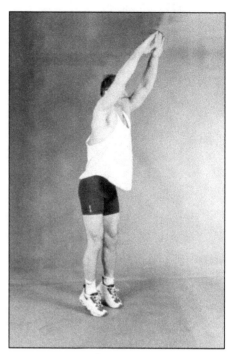

Fig 2-137

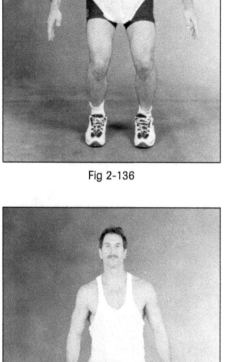

Fig 2-138

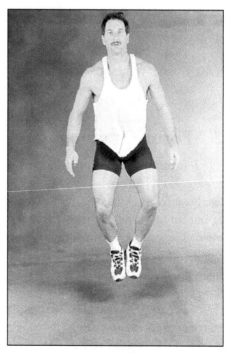

Fig 2-139

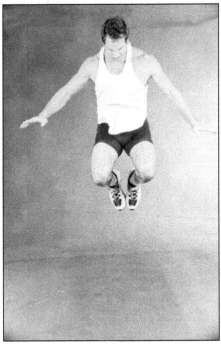

Fig 2-140

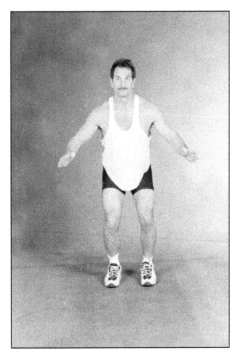

Fig 2-141

9. Increased power in your muscle contractions translate to increased power in your technique.

10. A faster technique is more powerful.

2.7 Forms Training

Tournament competitors are permitted to enter both sparring and forms for the same fee. I was too bulky to win forms consistently, but medalled regularly, probably because my master stressed the importance of forms. Smaller, compact competitors fare well, and so do those who can flip. It was encouraging however that judges occasionally rewarded the power, focus, and control of traditional martial arts forms.

Forms are a series of movements performed against imaginary opponents. The blocks, stances, and strikes within each form have remained intact for generations. Forms

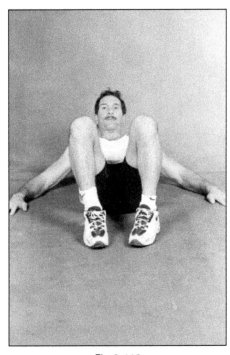

Fig 2-142

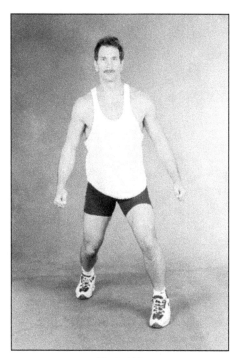

Fig 2-143

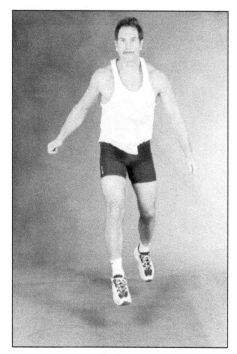

Fig 2-144

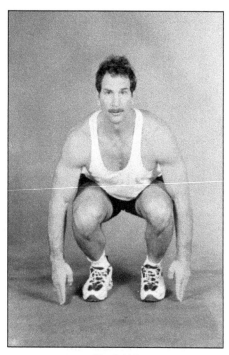

Fig 2-145

can be quite flowing and aesthetically pleasing, or can emphasize solid, basic techniques.

When you practice forms, visualize an opponent. Move quickly, powerfully, and precisely. As you block and strike, visualize your target. See and feel what you are doing. Without seeing and feeling your opponents, without imagining each technique, you are simply dancing without music.

The benefits of forms include enhanced concentration and improved conditioning. In addition, regular forms practice can train your reactions. Your body learns to use a technique without your conscious mind having to stop and think about it.

➲Tips on Forms

1. Stay Relaxed: Keep your body erect but at ease. With relaxation comes speed, power, balance, and good judgment.

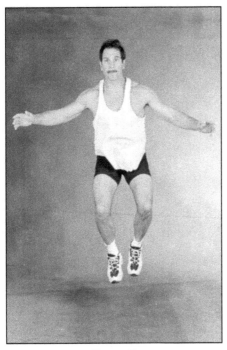

Fig 2-146

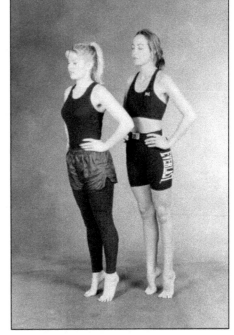

Fig 2-147

2. Focus your concentration on your imaginary opponent.

3. Stay level. When moving front and back or from side-to-side, keep your body on the same plane without bobbing up and down. Your knees should remain slightly bent as you slide smoothly on the balls of your feet.

4. Back straight, stomach in. Allow good posture to become a habit as you punch kick, strike, and block.

5. Exhale at the completion of each punch, kick, strike, and block.

6. Retract your punch or kick as quickly as you throw it.

7. Balance is important. Maintain your center of gravity over your hips.

8. Look in the direction of your movement, before you move.

9. Practice your forms in the dark.

10. Practice your forms in your head.

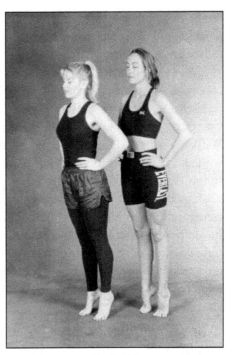

Fig 2-148

2.8 Balance

The legendary samurai Miyamoto Musashi once said, "Make your fighting stance your everyday stance, and make your everyday stance your fighting stance." Musashi survived more than sixty life-and-death duels. Hopefully you will not be required to fight to the death. Your altercations occur in the boardroom. Or in your kitchen. So, if you are standing, sitting, lying, leaning, or walking, you should be centered. No shifting, no wind-up. Pure balance.

Unnecessary physical tension detracts from balance. A static muscular contraction caused by stress interferes with your relaxed posture. Anxiety also affects your breathing, and therefore your body alignment. You may notice that worry increases tension in the muscles surrounding your sacrum in your lower back. Anxiety may debilitate your posture. You lose your equilibrium. A fret-filled day can bring you to your knees.

When you are stiff or tight, you're jerky and unsteady. You are at your best when you are relaxed, focused, and balanced. Balance means good posture, a neutral spine, and a firm stance. To find your neutral spine, stand with your heels, hips, shoulder blades, and head against a wall. Slip your hand in the space behind your low back, just above your hips. Your lower back (lumbar) area is curved slightly inward while your upper back (thoracic) area is counterbalanced outward. Sustain this posture throughout the day. A natural stance, with a neutral pelvis, demonstrates a relaxed countenance.

Balance is particularly important as you age. If you are off balance, it disturbs your mind in subtle ways. While balance obviously pertains to good posture, it also refers to your psychological profile. Correct posture is directly related to a relaxed, aware, ideal state of mind. The greater your awareness of your body, the better chance you have to be your best. Impeccable balance demonstrates a discipline of body and mind. You have a sense of power. Your movements are free and easy. You are sure of yourself, poised, and secure. You tend to have increased confidence. You have the ability to handle adverse situations with zeal.

Posture and balance allow you to move without wasted energy. Watch novice martial artists. Notice how they are tight and out of breath. Masters are graceful. They use only the muscles necessary to perform their techniques. There is no wasted energy. Every gesture has a reason.

To stand upright, without muscular effort, your body parts must be balanced around your center of gravity. Every movement you make, from kicking to blocking requires you to change your center of gravity. Your muscles exert force to re-establish equilibrium. The right and left sides of your body are almost symmetrical. The front and back halves of your body are too, allowing your spine to support you. A neutral posture prevents strain on ligaments and muscles.

Many times postural deviations are caused because yo do not maintain a neutral spine. For example, if you lean forward in your sparring stance day after day, week after week, postural imbalances develop. When you flex the spine in a forward lean, your disks are loaded unevenly. The ligaments in the back (posterior) of your spine become overstretched and create problems in your upper torso as well.

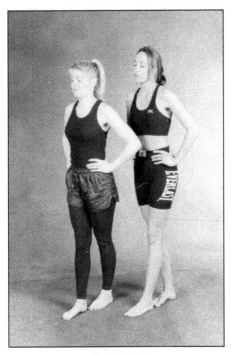

Fig 2-149

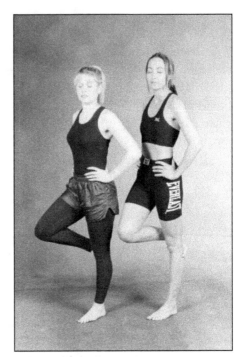

Fig 2-150

If you sit most of the day while eating, working, driving, and watching television, you inadvertently round your upper back and shorten or contract the muscles in your chest. This is exemplified in slumped shoulders, collapsed chest, and forward head. After years of assuming this unwieldy posture, it seems natural. When you try to change to a correct neutral spine, with your shoulders back, it feels stilted. That's why it's important to pay attention to your posture now. Make good posture, good balance, a habit.

Watch yourself practicing your martial arts in a mirror or on a video to help remedy your posture. Your deviation may be temporary if it was caused by muscle imbalance. To enhance alignment, sometimes specific stretching and strengthening exercises are necessary. You can improve your balance by using the following exercises.

Balance Exercises

Toe Hold: Rise on your toes, close your eyes and hold for twenty seconds (Figure 2-147).

Heel-to-Toe Hold: Place one foot in front of the other touching heel to toe. Close your eyes and hold for twenty seconds (Figure 2-148).

One-Legged Hold: Stand on one leg with your eyes closed for twenty seconds. Switch legs and repeat (Figure 2-149).

Heel Hold: Balance on your heels with your eyes closed for twenty seconds (Figure 2-150).

⟲Tips to Improve Your Balance

1. Keep your supporting knee slightly bent when performing any kicking technique.
2. Kick a target pad at full power while maintaining your center of gravity.
3. Punch without overextending your shoulder to maintain perfect balance.
4. Stand next to a wall and kick as many times as possible without dropping your leg. If you lose your balance, touch the wall to steady yourself.

CHAPTER 3

Mental Skills for Martial Artists

3.1 Everything Begins in Your Mind

At exactly seven P.M. our master lined us up. We dropped to our knees and faced a shrine and bowed in unison saying, "Please show me the way." At exactly nine P.M. we bowed out saying, "Thank you for showing me the way." These moments of silence showed our gratitude and cleared our minds in preparation for training.

Martial artists sometimes neglect the cognitive phase of their workouts. They spend hours physically preparing, but they spend little time in mental preparation. Training your mind is extremely important for exemplary achievement. Knowing when to turn it on will help you be your best.

Preparing for a martial arts tournament requires a tremendous amount of mental readiness. During idle moments your attention shifts to your upcoming contest. Your mind prepares your body for battle. Stomachs rumble, muscles tighten, and palms sweat. This "fight or flight response" is distressing to some. "Would be" competitors cannot handle tension. Their bodies become ill. Or they stumble and sprain ankles. Their sparring buddies say, "tough luck." They were simply not prepared to compete.

More likely, they may have been physically ready but not mentally fit. It is easy to exaggerate the caliber of adversaries or the magnitude of an event. Rather than viewing competition as win-lose, success-fail, approach each match as instruction. In a single tournament you will learn more about yourself than in six months of training.

Combating Competition Jitters

Competition brings out your best. Spectators increase your arousal, amplifying the urgency of your event. The better prepared you are, the more an audience will spur you on. For a few moments you are on the edge. It is electrifying. You may transcend your limits. It is an opportunity to be your best (Figure 3-1).

Emotions are a double edged sword. They increase your intensity but multiply your chances for error. Counterproductive feelings sabotage your performance. Defensiveness and negative emotions weaken you. Rage tears your game plan apart. During intense competition you may feel frustrated and experience antagonism. In anticipation of a tantrum, plan a response. Set limits on your emotional behavior. Promise yourself not to succumb. No matter how bad things become, acknowledge your opponent for issuing a challenge. The tougher he or she is, the more you will mature.

You have no control over your opponent's techniques or personality, so focus on your performance. If your rival displays malevolence, ignore it. When your opponent rages, use the misplaced energy to fuel your tenacity and courage. Develop a system. Emotions take a back seat. You cannot be enraged and centered at the same time.

Ask many top martial artists and they will admit performing optimally is mostly mental. Your mind programs your body for peak performance. Your body responds quickly when your brain is focused. In times of stress, like the remaining seconds before your event, it's easy to forget that you

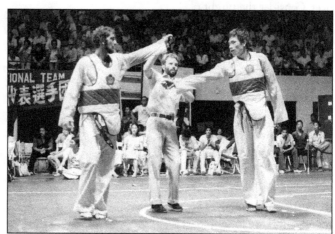

Fig 3-1

are in control. Here are some suggestions to help you calm competition nerves:

1. Recognize your symptoms of anxiety and ask yourself what could be so important to cause you to fret.
2. Understand that everyone gets butterflies.
3. Take a deep breath from your diaphragm and relax muscles that feel tense.
4. Visualize yourself appearing comfortably focused and prepared for your martial arts performance.
5. When your imagined performance begins, "see" everything going as planned.
6. Be spontaneous. A flexible attitude will allow you to relax, providing for a better performance.
7. Don't focus so much on yourself. Other people don't care as much about you as you do.
8. Empathize with the anxiety of your teammates. Help relieve their burden by relaxing.
9. Take control of yourself—be brave.

Your thoughts can provoke anxiety. Anxiety may lead to stress that intensifies poor martial arts performance. Breath observation will help you calm down. Breathe in through your nose by inhaling for a count of ten. Hold for five seconds and release your breath through your mouth for a count of five. Relax all of the muscles in your body. Focus only on your breathing. Follow your breath. Breathing is a very powerful relaxation technique.

Body/mind training is most effective when you are relaxed. Relaxation provides access to a state of mind that allows you to focus. Relaxation and proper concentration helps you maintain control. Replace apprehension with tenacity.

In a tournament you may compete for only a few minutes. The remainder of your time is spent waiting. Structure this respite to prepare for your subsequent bout. Begin thinking about your next opponent immediately. Don't exalt over victories until the tournament is over. Consider the plight of Dirk Jung, the 1977 defending heavyweight World Tae kwon do Champion from Germany. He beat me in the finals of the Asian Games in Taiwan just two months earlier. He was primed to win the 1979 World Championship in front of his home crowd in Stuttgart, Germany. The round before we fought, he had a ferocious fray with a Korean competitor. Jung

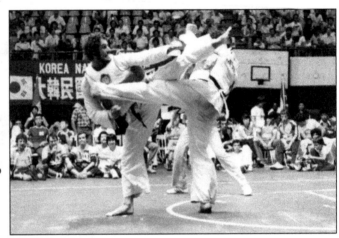

Fig 3-2

celebrated his conquest with a victory lap. He rejoiced and probably felt the battle was over, knowing that he had beat me once already. His body was in a recovery mode, leaving him flat. It was difficult for him to regroup and be his mental best for our fight. He lost (Figure 3-2).

➲Mental Tips

1. When anxiety strikes, monitor your muscles, and watch your breathing.

2. If you relax your muscles, your breathing will return to normal.

3. Supple muscles and deep rhythmic breathing allow you to handle anxiety.

3.2 Focus

Focus is an ambiguous term shrouded by mysticism. Some think focus leads to fulfillment and self-development. Psychologists say it is highly planned and controlled attention. As the brain intensifies its focus, it blocks out other stimuli, including pain. Martial artists believe that focus is the root of *Qi,* an inner strength. Everyone has *Qi* and the ability to focus it, but it is indeed difficult to develop. Focus allows practitioners to break bricks, lie on beds of nails, or land the killing blow in a duel to the death.

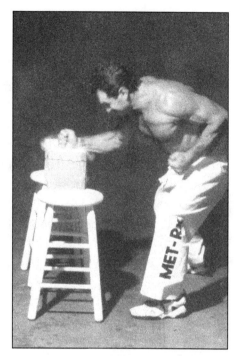

Whatever the goal, relax and concentrate. For instance, when you attempt to break a brick (Figure 3-3) or hit through an opponent, you must be relaxed, confident in your ability, and unhesitating in your commitment. When you are focused, time stands still. You may feel a profound sense of energized calm. Yet you are joyful and in control.

The ability to focus improves with practicing relaxation and concentration. If you are nervous, relax. The same ability to focus your arousal and attention are used to successfully lie on a bed of nails. You should be relaxed,

Fig 3-3

confident in your ability to support your weight evenly on the nails, and unflinching in your commitment to complete the action. You are in a special state of mind, and you are in control of this ideal performance state.

Practice focus in everything. Focus entirely on this book. Focus on the pitch you are hitting. Focus on the food you are eating. Focus on the person you are talking to. Give one hundred percent of your focus to all of your daily activities. Then the focus required to break a brick will come easy.

A relaxing method of practicing focus with a partner is called sticking hands:

1. Face your partner in a left side forward sparring position.
2. Close in so that your arms are touching.
3. Move your arms in a clockwise circle, keeping your elbows in.
4. Relax and keep constant contact with your partner's arms.
5. Close your eyes.
6. When you "feel" an opening, reach toward your partner's chest in a simulated strike.
7. Your partner should attempt to block in a circular motion without tension.
8. When your partner "feels" an opening, he/she reaches toward you as you attempt a smooth, circular block.
9. Continue sticking hands for three minutes.
10. Switch to a right side forward sparring position and continue for three minutes.

⊃Tips to Increase Focus

1. Focus is a combination of concentration and relaxation.
2. Speed comes from relaxation.
3. Concentrate your power into a small portion of your fist or foot (first two knuckles, knife edge, spear hand, elbow, heel, ball of foot).
4. Let your technique fly straight to the target.
5. Retract your technique as fast as your strike.
6. Exhale throughout the duration of your technique.
7. Mental focus feels calm, fearless, confident, and relaxed.
8. Focusing is fun.
9. What you think and how you act can increase or diminish your focus. Remain disciplined.
10. Focus gets better with practice.

3.3 Self Talk

There are no magic steps to a positive mental attitude. Simply look for the good. Become disciplined about what you say and think. Your thoughts affect how you feel. When unwanted images or thoughts slip into your consciousness use a counter-attack technique, or give yourself a quick pep talk. If you think about the punch that you failed to block, you will feel angry. If you think about a kick that scored, you will feel wonderful. You can reduce your nervousness, anxiety, and frustration by thinking positive thoughts. If you are talking yourself into training harder, be specific. Instead of saying "I ought to work with the heavy bag more, say "I will kick the heavy bag Tuesdays and Thursdays at six P.M." Our brains process what we say to ourselves. So talk to yourself, nicely.

Looking for the positive is important. Do not dwell on the negative. Some make a habit of complaining. It excites them. It is addicting. If you perceive a negative thought, let it go. Notice the bad, but don't focus it. Staying positive gives you power. Think about a positive event. How did you feel? Expand on your positive thoughts. Whatever you think about grows.

Do not permit a negative attitude to limit your martial arts performance. Hostility can affect your confidence and concentration. Transform fear or anger into focused energy. Start with relaxation. And then concentrate. Mental preparation is a skill. A disciplined mind does not come fast or easy, but if you keep at it, you will succeed.

⊃Tips on Positive Self Talk

1. Commit to becoming disciplined about what you let yourself think.
2. Become aware of the type of thoughts that flow through your mind.
3. Set thinking goals. Your goals should reflect your purpose in martial arts.

4. If you find yourself saying negative thoughts to yourself, immediately reverse them to positive thoughts.

5. Practice positive thinking all of the time.

3.4 Pain Management

My most severe martial arts injury happened en route to the Pre-World Games in Taiwan. Sitting for eighteen hours straight hastened the growth of a pilonidal cyst on my tailbone, requiring surgery when I returned to the United States.

Sometimes you must experience discomfort to succeed. Talk yourself through it. You can boost yourself. What do you say to yourself? Sit against a wall with your thighs parallel to the floor. What does your brain tell you? What do you tell your brain?

Do you strive to meet the status quo? Are you working hard to be mediocre? At some point we come to a fork in the road. We can merely choose to survive, or we can decide to achieve our personal martial arts potential. To reach a lofty goal, pain and discomfort must be overcome.

Before we proceed you should understand the difference between "bad pain" and "good pain." "Bad pain" is the kind that results from injury, whether it's a pulled muscle, a strain, broken bones, etc. Whenever you feel pain from an injury, stop what you are doing. That pain is a signal from your body telling you that something needs to be fixed. It is possible to overcome the pain of an injury, but in the long run you are only doing yourself more harm.

"Good pain" is the discomfort of intense training that stops when you stop. Mastering your art requires this kind of pain. Almost all aspects of martial arts training push the pain barrier. If you never take the opportunity to endure, you miss out. Pain is natural and can be positive, albeit potentially uncomfortable. The origin of pain is not at issue, controlling it is.

What can you do? Relax. Get used to it. Pain makes you a better martial artist. Face discomfort. Learn about it, and pain won't seem severe. Accept pain for what it is and handle it. Without pain there is no accomplishment or real happiness. Pain is uncomfortable, but it is not the end of the world.

Pain can be overridden. Harvard scientists gave morphine to one group of patients after surgery and sugar pills to another group. Seventy-five percent of the placebo group felt the same relief as if they had taken the morphine.

The body deals with pain in different ways. During my black belt test, I was punched in the spleen. Moments after the test severe pain forced my knees to my chest, and I was rushed to the hospital. Receptors transmitted pain to my brain during the test, but there were other signals as well. Sparring and forms drowned out the agony in my side. At the hospital, however, there was no stimulation to compete so pain took center stage.

I have witnessed broken noses and ribs. I watched a man fighting while his arm was hanging dislocated from his shoulder. He tucked it into his uniform and continued.

Another fighter limped through three, three-minute rounds and later X-rays determined he had been fighting on a broken leg.

According to Melzack's Gate Control Theory, thousands of pain signals come together across nerve fibers that meet between the spinal cord and the brain. This traffic jam of signals allows some signals to get through while others wait. Some never make it.

The pain messages that reach the brain may be controlled. The mind can magnify pain or sublimate it. Pain signals can scream so loud they drown out rational thought. Or those howls of agony can be transformed to shouts of joy. The first few days of a serious training schedule are intense. Muscle fibers split and joints ache. You can choose to interpret these signals as debilitating or ecstatic. Your ability to handle pain is what sets you apart from also-rans and spectators. Approach pain with courage. Deal with it on your terms. Handle pain one step at a time.

3.5 Rhythm

During the Pan American Games, I called my teammates together between rounds to sing my favorite tune, "Celebration." I carried the rhythm into the ring and fought my best. Music was my motivation.

Research has demonstrated that music can affect concentration, endurance, muscle tension, blood pressure, heart rate, and breathing. Music increases positive emotions and lifts spirits by stimulating neurochemical changes associated with healing. Feeling joyful may be triggered by listening to upbeat, fast tempos with simple harmonies and flowing rhythms.

According to the Aerobics and Fitness Association of America, training to music can bring good health, motivation, and harmony. Several studies have demonstrated the benefits of training to music. Exercisers at Ohio State confirmed that they felt less perceived exertion when they worked out to music. Another investigation reported in the Journal of Sports Medicine and Physical Fitness showed that music makes exercise seem less difficult, allowing the participant to continue longer.

Nobody expected me to win the 1979 National AAU Taekwondo Championships—even I considered myself a long shot. Between each fight I found a quiet place and listened to the sound track from *Superman*, the movie. I imagined myself strong, powerful, and fast. I was confident and fought better than ever, beating the defending national champion in the finals to qualify for international competition.

⮁Tips on Music Selection

1. Use music that makes you feel confident, calm, energetic, and relaxed.
2. Use your music regularly to summon feelings that you need during martial arts training.
3. Make a tape and keep a tape player around during your practice sessions.
4. When you feel strong and confident from listening to your music selections, visualize yourself as an unbeatable martial artist.

3.6 Discipline

When I returned to the United States I couldn't find any martial arts schools, so I taught a seven A.M. class at my high school. Teaching punches, kicks, strikes, and blocks forced me to analyze each move. I became a better martial artist because in teaching others I refined my technique.

About sixty percent of those who begin training quit within the first six months. The most common excuse is boredom. Endlessly practicing the same basic techniques is boring for some, but not for the disciplined. Although the bored and the disciplined train at the same place and at the same time, they are opposite. Energy level, motivation, and intensity are obviously dissimilar. Bored combatants are mindlessly throwing hands and feet; their disciplined counterparts are punching and kicking imaginary opponents. Casual students slack off at the first sign of discomfort; disciplined trainers begin at this point. The bored train the least. The disciplined clear their minds and focus. They are in the moment. The disciplined are rarely bored. If everyone were disciplined, all would master their art.

Martial arts are so multifaceted that boredom is not an option. Disciplined training is life. Techniques are half your training. The other half is mental and spiritual. Tap into your samurai role model, but focus on your goal. Creating a clear mental picture of your goal makes training easy. Minute to minute, day to day, month to month, and year to year goals are reached, and new ones sought. Whether preparing for a tournament or improving self defense, kicking higher, punching harder, perfecting that takedown, moving faster, staying calmer are but a few goals you can strive for. No two workouts are alike because each fulfills a different promise of perfection.

Your master may help provide you with the motivation to throw those last three kicks. He psyches you up when you feel weak and tired. A training partner is also useful, serving as a crutch to force you to work hard when you'd rather be a couch potato. But no matter if you have the best instructor or most reliable workout partner, you won't get far in martial arts if you lack self-discipline. Teamwork is fine, but you've got to be motivated on your own if you're going to succeed. The search for improvement starts from within. Disciplined training is a path to a new sense of self.

Elite martial artists discipline both their bodies and minds. In many martial arts there are no time-outs, substitutions, or coaching during competition to give you a breather. Fighters spend hours alone with their thoughts. Periodically they examine their choices. They determine if they struggle to reach someone else's goal. Or search themselves to discover the reasons they do what they do.

Look back on your life. List your accomplishments. Any worthwhile achievement required perseverance. Finishing school, playing a musical instrument, or attaining a black belt required discipline. Draw upon your past challenges to shape your future.

"Building your body can be achieved only when your mind has been disciplined." says Lao Tzu. Get hooked on disciplined training. An afternoon of lounging can't beat a spirited workout. At first, it is easier to forego exercise and watch television. Some people crave alcohol or gambling, but working out is better than any drug. The secret is to convince yourself that martial arts are play. How can spending hours punching and kicking be pleasurable? It's fun if you know when to start, and finish. Set guidelines as to how much time to devote to activity.

Disciplined exercise requires you to set aside just a few minutes each day. Maintain your program until it is routine. Always look forward to your activity. Never burn out. If priorities conflict, be flexible. Once training is a habit, it's easy.

Set short and long term goals. Begin with baby steps. Progress gradually. In six months you will become accustomed to your program. Increase your intensity no more than five percent for a given workout. If you are too vigorous your body will revolt. With proper planning however, you can discipline yourself to do almost anything.

Discipline is living every moment without regret. Some think pleasure is partying all night. But true happiness requires discipline. Find your discipline and you will discover the martial artist within.

⊃Tips on Improving Discipline

1. Train daily with a clear, uncluttered mind.
2. Spend a few moments in breathing meditation.
3. With each technique, visualize your imaginary opponent.
4. Use a mirror to check your form.
5. Look forward to a slight bit of discomfort.
6. Set goals for your training such as becoming faster or stronger.
7. Use a bag or striking pad to evaluate your power.
8. When you reach a goal, set a new one.
9. Practice zeroing in on your goals.
10. Visualize your goals and the training required to reach them.
11. Off of the practice floor, daydream about martial arts. On the practice floor, fulfill your dream.

3.7 Burning Desire

Every Friday was clean-up night in our training hall. White belts and masters shared stories while busily scrubbing floors and cleaning windows. The camaraderie was essential in creating a family atmosphere in our normally strict and formal *dojang*.

Ancient wisdom suggests to live in moderation. But too much moderation leads to mediocrity. Be adventurous. Make a wish list of long term martial arts goals: Win the World Championships, perform exquisite form, become an action hero. Break these into smaller and easier to handle segments: Win the Regional Championships, practice forms daily, make your own martial arts video. Focus on arriving at each intermediate destination. Don't immerse yourself in the final goal until you are well on your way. By breaking down the ultimate challenge into manageable parts, you will enjoy success one day at a time.

Sometimes there may be no goal. No tournament. Nobody to impress. No motivation. Try something different. Analyze a baseball game. Play tennis. Meditate. Pray. Tend your garden. Any activity is art. Love your art no matter your skill level. Your *sensei,* coach, or teacher cannot motivate you. Motivation comes from within. Some have a burning desire to improve while others do well to show up. Breaks are natural, and moderation fuels motivation over the long haul; obsessiveness does not. If you really hate to train, ask yourself: a. Are you working out too hard? b. Are you working out too much? c. Do you feel alone? Regardless of your level of motivation, you can excel if you adhere to the following program:

A. Month 1: Make your training a habit.

1. Do not miss any classes for your first month.
2. Clear your schedule to be sure of no conflicts.
3. If you dread going to class, tell yourself you can quit after a month.
4. Reward yourself after each class with a cold drink.
5. Practice your strengths, go through the motions of your weaknesses.
6. Make an effort to develop friendships with other students.
7. After a month, evaluate your progress.
8. If you despise the notion of attending class, quit.

B. Month 2: Enjoy your training.

1. Go out of your way to introduce yourself to new members of the class.
2. During a break, ask beginners if they need any help.
3. Set training goals based on your potential.
4. Make it a point to cordially ask advanced students questions about your progress.
5. Still your wandering mind; practice focusing your concentration.
6. Practice proper form without concern for intensity.
7. Show respect and congeniality to all of your classmates.

C. Month 3: Put your heart in your art.

1. Each time you attend class work on a specific goal (e.g. speed, intensity, flexibility).
2. Put your heart and soul into your training.
3. Work on your weaknesses as well as your strengths.
4. Give one hundred percent of yourself to each of your workouts.
5. Ask your instructor to help you reach your potential.
6. Practice the finer points and details of your movements.
7. Develop your inner strength through proper relaxation and focus.
8. Become an artist. Individualize each technique to fit your body type.
9. Attend tournaments to evaluate your progress.
10. Never stop learning.

D. Month 4: Re-evaluate your goals.

1. If your initial goal was to become world champion, but you can only train twice a week for half an hour, choose to become master of your art.
2. Help a fellow student improve a technique during each workout.
3. Encourage two students by telling them they have improved.
4. Don't worry about your motivation. You are hooked.

⤵Motivation Tips

1. Search yourself for the reason you train in the martial arts: physical, mental, spiritual, self-defense, competition, affiliation, endorphins, relaxation, discipline, or self-confidence.
2. Enjoy your training. Stay in the moment.
3. Be the best you can be. Each of your techniques can be improved.
4. Remind yourself that benefits of martial arts training include a better physique, increased ability to handle stress, improved health, enhanced concentration, and an interconnected mind/body.

3.8 Overtraining

Many work hard at the martial arts, training for a specific purpose or event. If they don't see improvement, they try harder. The harder they try, the more tension and anxiety they feel.

It's easy to eat, sleep, and drink martial arts. You can stretch, practice punches and kicks, cross-train with weights/aerobics, and watch training videos. There seems to be a point of diminishing returns to excessive training, however. Some enthusiasts train so frequently they develop overuse injuries. They think they must push beyond their normal limits to get to the next level. Elbows, knees, and backs simply wear out. Recent research suggests that immune systems become impaired with too much training, leading to colds, flu, and other infections.

Others burn out psychologically. Their lives revolve around martial arts. Relationships and jobs suffer. All they can think about is training or competition. Training is like drinking a glass of wine. A little bit with each meal is fine, but too much and they become alcoholics.

Mastering your art is a way of life, but there is more to life than training. There is no specific standard to how much a martial artist can take. Everything you do, from eating and sleeping to socializing, can be placed under the martial arts umbrella. Know when to leave the training hall. Pushing too hard leads to a breakdown of the toughening process. Alternate heavy and light workouts to achieve peak performance. If you are out on a date and all you can think about is an upcoming tournament, you may be out of balance. If you think you are out of balance, consider the following questions:

1. In five years, what do you plan to be doing?
2. Who are the most important people in your life?
3. What is your purpose on this earth?
4. When you leave the world, what would you have people say about you?
5. Who is your role model?
6. What would you do tomorrow if you had one week to live?
7. If you could see your family and friends at your funeral, what would they be saying about you?

Signs of overtraining include:

1. Elevated heart rate. If your heart rate is higher than normal when you awaken, you may be overtraining.
2. Negative attitude. Inadequate recovery from training may lead to listlessness.
3. Weight loss. Overtraining can lead to muscle loss and weakness.
4. Lack of recovery. After a tournament you may recover slowly if you have over-trained because your immune system is depressed.
5. Loss of interest. Overtraining leads to boredom and lack of commitment.
6. Fatigue. Overtraining causes fatigue from even a mild training session.
7. Injury. Overtraining may cause overuse injuries and muscle pain.

The hard part is distinguishing between overtraining and laziness. Balance of mind, body, and spirit is crucial for peak performance. Discuss it with experienced classmates or your instructor. Listen to your body. If you fear you are on the verge of overtraining, you probably are.

CHAPTER 4

Relaxation, Meditation, & Imagery for Peak Performance

4.1 Breathing

My 6 month old breathes from her nose and fills the lower lobes of her lungs. Only when she cries does she mouth breathe, huffing and puffing from her upper chest. When adults are nervous they mouth breathe from their upper chests. Lack of attention to our air flow likens us to a hyperventilating, scared rabbit.

When you experience stress and anxiety, your body prepares for a crisis. Blood is quickly transported to your muscles for fight or flight. Your blood pressure increases and so does your heart rate. To get the oxygen you need, and to expel carbon dioxide more quickly, you breathe faster and more erratically from your chest. Exhaling carbon dioxide too quickly disturbs your blood pH. This keeps your blood from efficiently getting oxygen to your brain, muscles, and organs. When you inhale-exhale impulsively, you hyperventilate. And if you are anxious all day long, you may be in a constant state of hyperventilation. You may be hyperventilating at this very moment.

The anxiety and stress that cause hyperventilation are not related strictly to a tough sparring session or pre-competition jitters. Any type of stress or anxiety—at work, home, anywhere—can trigger this response in your body. Some estimates suggest that sixty to ninety percent of medical ailments are stress related. Therefore, your martial arts training and your overall health will benefit from becoming aware of your breathing and learning to breathe more efficiently.

If you find yourself in a stressful situation, take a deep breath from your belly. Focus on your breathing. This short circuits your sympathetic nervous system and lessens your stress reaction. Automatically your heart rate and blood pressure drop. Just by altering your attention, you decrease your anxiety. There is no room for negativity. Pain patients use breathing techniques to lessen their discomfort and increase relaxation. You can do it too.

The lower lobes of your lungs are below your chest. Breathe deeply and allow air to fill this area. This is diaphragmatic breathing. Muscle tension, especially tight abdominals, constrict your diaphragm. So does holding your stomach in to appear svelte. Wearing a tight belt teaches you to breathe improperly too.

Your lower lungs inflate with less effort than your upper lungs. But you probably do not take advantage of this. Count your inhalations. You probably inhale about twenty times per minute. Try taking in more air with each breath. Fill your lungs. This allows you to breathe slower and more smoothly. Breathing smoothly helps stabilize your blood pH. Belly breathers average eight to fourteen inhalations per minute.

Relaxed, focused breathing builds lung capacity, eases stress, energizes your body, and enhances your rhythm. Learn to breathe from your diaphragm instead of your chest. To get the feel of it, try this simple exercise. Lie on your back. Place your left hand on your chest and your right hand on your stomach. Inhale from your nose, deeply and slowly, for five seconds, focusing on lowering your diaphragm. Let the air fill your lower, central, and upper chest, in that order. Then take about seven seconds to exhale slowly through your mouth by raising your diaphragm. Only your right hand should move as you breathe deeply from your abdomen. Diaphragmatic breathing allows you to get more oxygen to your working muscle. Notice how muscles in your body spontaneously relax. You can also do this exercise when you are standing and sitting. It's a great way to relieve stress and tension, energize you, and you can do it anywhere.

Practice focused breathing whenever you can. It helps to decrease anxiety and sharpens your concentration. Use focused breathing between rounds of a bout to increase your energy. Take complete breaths from your nose during practice, and each respiratory perfusion become longer, deeper, and slower; this allows your body to remain relaxed, even under extreme stress. Conclusion—breathe from your tummy, always.

4.2 Relaxation

Stress in modern times tends to be chronic. The pace of our lives is so fast that car phones, computers, and fax machines allow us to work day and night. Our bodies are able to handle stress, but not all of the time. We must be able to respond to stress, and also know how to relax at will. Ideally, we should learn to cope with a stressor, and then relax.

Are you aware of your own feelings of anxiety? Do you walk around with unnecessary tension in your muscles? If so, take a deep breath from your diaphragm as explained in the previous section. Exhale, and allow tension in any part of your body to be released. If you are tired, a deep breath can make you more alert. When you learn the difference between tension and relaxation you will perform all your martial arts activities more effectively. Relaxing your muscles makes you faster. Trying too hard increases muscle tension and stiffness, slowing down your performance. Let your techniques happen with relaxed but concentrated force.

When you claim you do not have time to relax, that is when you need it the most. But you cannot force yourself to relax. Relaxation will happen if you let it. Here's an easy way to practice relaxation. It only takes a minute (literally), but if you enjoy it and find it helpful, you can increase the time.

⟳Mini-Relaxation Technique

1. Close your eyes and consciously relax your muscles (ten seconds).
2. Breathe from your diaphragm. Focus on your breath (twenty seconds).
3. See, feel, and experience yourself in your favorite resting place (thirty seconds).
4. Slowly open your eyes.

I recommend doing a relaxation technique about twenty minutes each day. Try to find your own special relaxation place. Soon you will enjoy deep levels of relaxation other than during your designated relaxation time. You can learn to relax anywhere, anytime.

Another way to release stress and anxiety is a Body Awareness Check. Oftentimes, we unconsciously hold ourselves in tight, uncomfortable positions. For instance, driving in traffic may cause you to tense your shoulders, tighten your belly, even grit your teeth. Sitting for long periods may cause you to slouch or hunch your shoulders. Make it a habit to run through this Body Awareness Checklist several times a day.

⟳Body Awareness Checklist

1. Monitor your present level of anxiety (muscles, breathing, mental activity).
2. Is your anxiety level high, low, or just right?
3. If it is high, take a deep breath from your diaphragm. Exhale and let all of the tension flow out of your body.
4. Adjust your body so that you are alert without tension.

As a graduate student in sport psychology, I signed up for a hypnosis class. My sixty-five year old instructor was taking us through a relaxation-induction technique. She asked us to lie on the floor as she performed a hypnotic induction: "Close your eyes, breathe from your diaphragm, focus on your breathing so that every time you exhale you go deeper and deeper...Cough, Belch, Belch, Cough, Cough, Cough, Belch." My classmates and I awakened with a start, attempting to stifle our hysterical laughter. That lesson taught me that humor is also good for relaxation. A good belly laugh releases anxiety.

Relaxing isn't loafing or laziness. It's moving without tension. You can be relaxed and alert at the same time. When you are tight, your brain thinks something is wrong. So stay relaxed, and keep in mind that peak performance begins with inner calm.

Of course, it is possible to become too relaxed. During the World Championships, I was in the locker room practicing my relaxation exercise. I was suddenly aroused as the loudspeaker blared, "Last call, Seabourne, U.S.A." I had fallen asleep on the locker room bench.

Personalize your relaxation techniques to meet your needs. You might take a deep breath, or stretch, or close your eyes for a few minutes. You could daydream about the beach, or practice diaphragm breathing. Or imagine yourself as a Zen monk, living quietly in the mountains. Whatever works for you, do it.

4.3 Meditation

As a high school student I saw an advertisement for a free introductory lecture to a course called Transcendental Meditation (T.M.). The proponents of the course claimed that within five to eight years of training, a student would reach cosmic consciousness. The T.M. seminar leader was graceful and he coughed silently. His movements were extremely slow and deliberate. I wondered if he had reached enlightenment. I raised my hand and inquired, "Sir, have you reached cosmic consciousness?" He looked surprised and faced me sternly saying, "It's not me we're concerned with." I realized he had not.

I practiced T.M. everyday for five years and never reached enlightenment. In fact, the year I quit doing T.M., I was a senior at Penn State University. An acquaintance of mine had also taken the T.M. course. I asked him to tell me his mantra. He said, "No, if I tell you my mantra, my instructor said it wouldn't work for me anymore." I said, "I'll tell you mine if you tell me yours." We had been given the same mantra—'ing.'

Twenty years later, after marriage and children, I picked up where I left off and once again enjoy the benefits of relaxed concentration. Sometimes I have a baby crawling all over me, or I do it in a boring meeting, and often ten minutes is my limit, but I continue to reap the rewards of quiet meditation. My relaxed concentration carries over to the rest of my day.

Meditation is not hard, or time consuming. It is simply focusing on what you are doing. When was the last time you watched a good movie? Was it so intense that you were unconscious of your surroundings? Were you so engrossed that you forgot you were hungry, thirsty, or needed to go to the bathroom? That is a striking example of the power of focus.

Meditation can help you develop good focus. You can make every action or thought a process of meditation. Immerse yourself in any activity. Let distractions enter one ear and proceed out the other.

Meditate anytime, anywhere. Meditate while waiting in line, riding in a car (not while driving though), or sitting quietly with your eyes closed. Extend your meditation time from seconds to minutes. If you enjoy your meditation you will continue.

Meditation allows you to focus your attention. Concentrate on your studies, martial arts, or social interactions. Devote your attention to any movement, idea, or project that is worthwhile.

Stare at something—a plant, tree, book, whatever. Focus your attention on this object for two minutes. Then close your eyes. Bring back the object in your mind's eye.

See it, with your eyes closed. Let your visualization become your focus. This also, is meditation. The object of your meditation can be prayer, martial arts, or a bowl of cereal. It does not matter. Enjoy it.

Meditation is non-competitive. Do not say, "I must meditate for twenty minutes, or I have failed." Instead, let yourself meditate for as long or as little as you want to. Meditate on any physical, mental, or spiritual thing. The process is important, not the goal.

Meditation becomes easier with practice. Meditation is a skill, the same as a punch. The more you rehearse, the better you become. But don't worry if you are a slow learner. Concern about your progress will impede your improvement.

I have been fortunate to study a variety of meditation strategies from instructors all over the world. In my experience, the one most beneficial to martial arts training is based on the Relaxation Response developed by Herbert Benson, M.D. The Relaxation Response is a relaxed and focused mind-set you hope to achieve both in and out of the training hall. Some folks tap their fingers and fidget to ease tension. Others meditate. Dr. Benson, who is a Harvard trained cardiologist, has extolled the advantages of repeating a monosyllabic phrase to reduce stress and improve well-being. His studies with transcendental meditators demonstrated that a few minutes of quiet repetition can manifest tremendous physiological gains.

Find a quiet place to sit and relax. Close your eyes and breathe from your diaphragm. Each time you exhale, say the word "one" under your breath. Say "one" whenever you think of it. Whenever any thoughts or sounds disturb you, let the distractions go in one ear and out the other and go back to "one." When twenty minutes have passed, slowly open your eyes.

As you concentrate, keep your body at ease. Your breathing and heart rate will slow, and your blood pressure will decrease. After a while there will be no thoughts. Nothing. Soon you are what you are doing—relaxed and focused.

Each meditative experience is different, however. Sometimes I focus deeply and sincerely for the entire twenty minutes, and other times I awaken from a deep sleep forty-five minutes later. Some days dinner was foremost on my mind, and some days there is nothing but "one." If you don't have twenty minutes, do a mini-strategy. Instead of missing a session, do five minutes. It's better than nothing, and will help you maintain your practice.

At Penn State I was a subject in an experiment where I was required to watch a movie while electrodes measured my muscle activity and galvanic skin response. The movie began innocently, but without warning a man was impaled by a two-by-four. Meditators (me included) showed less muscle tension and a greater galvanic skin response than non-meditators, confirming that they manage stress more effectively.

An important part of meditation is breathing. Deep rhythmic breathing is your key to success. The diaphragm breathing described in section 4.1 is also useful for meditation. In addition to the physical benefits, diaphragm breathing can provide a focus for your mind and improve your concentration.

You can meditate while lying down, sitting, even standing (Figures 4-1, 4-2, and 4-3). Take a deep breath from your diaphragm, then exhale. Relax. Focus on your

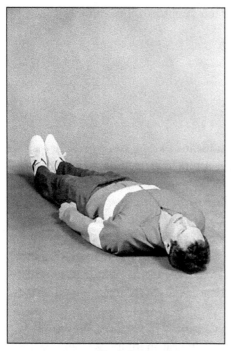

Fig 4-1

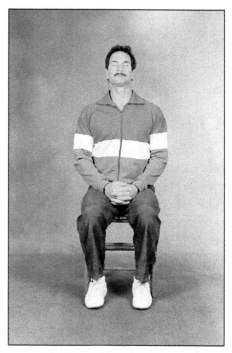

Fig 4-2

breathing. Let nothing distract or disturb you; just breathe. Concentrate on "one" or on your breathing. If thoughts or sounds interfere, notice them but let them go. Close this book, close your eyes, and continue relaxing. After five minutes, slowly come out of your relaxed state. How do you feel? Close your eyes and continue meditating for twenty minutes.

➲Tips on Meditation

1. Find a quiet room.
2. Lower the lights.
3. Loosen clothing.
4. Sit in an upright posture so that you don't doze off.
5. Meditate before meals so that you are alert.
6. Come out of your relaxation very slowly.
7. Put your answering machine on and use ear plugs if necessary.

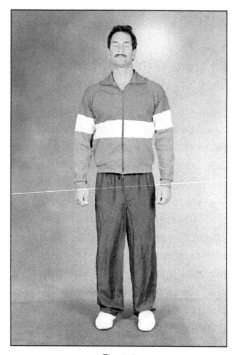

Fig 4-3

8. If you don't have twenty minutes, do it for ten minutes, or five minutes.

9. Try to meditate at least once a day.

10. Consistency is important.

4.4 Imagery

Train your mind to become focused at idle moments. During those twilight stages before sleep, and as you awaken, imagine you have achieved your goals. I visualize myself enjoying my family. Then I feel myself attacking and defending with unstoppable endurance. Finally, I see myself helping others reach their goals. You can focus on your martial arts while listening to a boring lecture or driving. Be careful not to careen off the side of a mountain while you practice your forms in your imagination.

Can you visualize a triangle? A square? Your own body as if you were looking into a mirror? Can you imagine the way you would like to feel after one year of serious martial arts training? See yourself, feel yourself, experience yourself having achieved your martial arts goals.

Humans appear to be the only organism with the ability to visualize. We can send blood away from or to certain areas of our bodies to help heal an injury. We can imagine ourselves performing a technique, which will then aid our martial arts in 'real life.' We can disassociate from the pain of a dentist's drill by picturing ourselves in a peaceful scene. And we can affect our bodies at the cellular level to strengthen our immune system.

Imagery With Your Eyes Wide Open

Before we go on to a few imagery exercises, I'd like to share this personal story about the power of visualizations.

At the World Championships, my first fight was with the representative from Morocco, and if I won I would fight the Frenchman. With no medal round in sight, my next bout would be the German defending world champion, fighting in his home country. My first two fights were action-packed as I won on a technical knockout and a unanimous decision.

Moments prior to my third fight, my coach told me to foul the German in an attempt to be disqualified so the U.S. team would not lose face. I disregarded my coach and went on to narrowly defeat the German. It seemed a gold medal was assured. I won my semi-final bout in an uneventful slug-fest with the Australian representative. The gold medal round began with my opponent and me exhausted from a long day of punches and kicks. At the end of round one, I had the edge. Then the unimaginable occurred; I fouled my opponent from the Netherlands by punching him in the face, sending him sprawling to the canvas. The doctor stepped in the ring to check his condition. At this point, the referees called a meeting, which continued for twenty minutes. They concluded that I was to be disqualified. My Dutch opponent continued to feign pain, but when he was awarded the gold he jumped for joy with no trace of injury.

My coach told me to punch the German competitor in the face because he thought I had no chance to win. I visualized myself committing the foul, but could not actually go through with the act. Ironically, two bouts later I unconsciously punched my opponent to the face. Your visualizations can come true. So be careful what you visualize.

My college physiology instructor made me a relaxation-imagery audio tape designed to improve my martial arts performance. While listening to the tape before bedtime, I imagined myself punching and kicking, winning one bout after another.

I practiced imagery while working at a job engraving name tags. As my eyes and hands unconsciously copied a template, my mind was immersed in the world of martial arts. I imagined myself punching and kicking in tournaments. I conjured up a clear picture, concentrating on color and detail, sometimes questioning myself about the texture of the floor. If I visualized I was about to be knocked out by a ruthless attack, I mentally counter-attacked.

There are two ways to practice imagery to improve your martial arts performance: external imagery and internal imagery. External imagery is when you "see" yourself practicing a technique, as if watching on television. Internal imagery utilizes your ability to "feel" yourself performing.

Recent research suggests that imagery is most effective when practiced from the internal perspective. This is not surprising because internal imagery may enhance innervation (stimulation) of the proper nerve to muscle pathways. When performing internal imagery you may actually feel your muscles twitch as they respond to your mental machinations.

Here is an exercise you can do to practice internal imagery. The exercise focuses on a side kick, but you can perform internal imagery exercises with any of your techniques. The main point is to stay relaxed as you visualize the technique, and feel it happening. Imagery is most successful through repetition and concentration.

Internal Imagery Training

1. Clear your mind.
2. Look down and slightly to your left side.
3. "Feel" your left leg cocking itself into a perfect side kick fold position.
4. Imagine extending your leg from your hip until you sense that it has "locked" into a perfect side kick position.
5. Bring your foot back to your knee.
6. Set it down.
7. Practice ten repetitions of your internal side kick.

Research

Studies show that training and practice with internal imagery can improve your martial arts performance. Research that Bob Weinberg and I conducted at the University of North Texas demonstrated:

1. Relaxation and imagery combined was more beneficial for martial arts students than either relaxation or imagery alone.

2. Martial arts students who practiced relaxation and imagery ten minutes each day performed significantly better than those who were exposed to the technique moments prior to their performance.

3. When we individualized the mental techniques to the needs of the martial arts students, they performed better than a control group.

4. That instructor-guided imagery was no more effective than self-guided imagery. Results showed no significant differences in martial arts performance between the self-guided group and the instructor-guided group.

5. That individualizing cognitive techniques to the needs of the students significantly improved their martial arts performance.

Imagery and Modeling

Imagine Jackie Chan evading an attacker's thrust by easily jumping back and executing a double flip to an adjacent rooftop. These antics are commonplace in martial arts flicks. But can you learn something from watching them? The answer is yes and no. Regardless of how many flying double back flips you watch, there will probably be no transfer of skill from the silver screen to your own double-back flipping capabilities. However, some martial arts movies have a great deal to offer in the way of technical excellence. Visualize Van Damme performing a roundhouse kick. Simply by viewing his incredible speed, timing, and efficient technique, you might be inspired to train just a little bit harder, and subsequently improve your own speed, timing, and efficiency.

⮑Modeling Tips

1. Whether you see it in a martial arts movie, a tournament or a seminar, make a mental picture of a perfect movement that you have witnessed.

2. Review the move over and over in your mind's eye.

3. Use as many of your senses as possible. Try to "feel" the move as if you were actually performing it. "Hear" the sound of the technique as it snaps through the air.

4. Physically shadow box the movement as you visualize it.

5. Finally, physically practice the movement.

6. Practice both physically and mentally until your physical technique approaches the perfection of your mental ideal.

7. Establish routines.

8. Describe yourself as powerful and fast.

4.5 Mind and Body

In martial arts, the process is at least as important as the product. Perfecting the movements is art. The daily ritual of repetitive practice sharpens the body and mind. Spending hours honing movements, bending knees, and executing technique, can be meaningful, or painfully boring. Martial artists who disdain practice may achieve a modicum of success, but practice makes champions.

Elite martial artists spend hours whittling their bodies into condition. Stronger, more agile athletes who have more endurance are superior competitors. Their commitment to training is strengthened by daily short term achievements. To become champions, a disciplined mental and physical practice schedule is a normal part of their everyday routine.

The skills and exercises discussed in this chapter and chapter three should be a regular part of your workout. Your mind and body are intertwined. To achieve your best, you've got to keep both in top condition. Following are some reminders about the skills you've learned from chapters three and four.

⊃Psychological Skills Training Tips

1. Psychological skills must be practiced, not just read about.
2. Psychological skills improve over time.
3. Psychological skills are improved in response to pressurized, stressful situations.
4. Different psychological skills work for different situations.
5. Psychological skills training is a long-term process, measured in months, not days.
6. Use your psychological skills, or lose them.

CHAPTER 5

Training Outside Your Martial Arts School

5.1 Training Anytime, Anywhere!

While a student at Penn State I played on the varsity tennis team. When we traveled to tournaments, I would play my match (and usually lose), then I'd practice martial arts until my teammates were done. Soon I was spending more time practicing martial arts then tennis. I entered martial arts tournaments on weekends and returned to my studies with a swollen nose and black eyes. I didn't win much, but I was improving.

You can practice your art anytime, anywhere. With as little as six square feet you can punch, kick, block, strike, and practice your forms. I shadow-sparred in hotel rooms and airports, kicked in bus stations, target trained on tennis courts, and practiced forms on racquetball courts.

Training alone will give you the opportunity to practice details. Focus on the angle of your foot. Notice if your hand is twisted to forty-five degrees. Check your stances. Address problems you may overlook in class. Refine your movements until they are near perfect. It doesn't matter who's around. Some will stop and stare, but most will go about their business. Just keep in mind that a humble spirit attracts few onlookers, but showing off brings trouble. Challengers test an arrogant spirit. Be concerned with your proficiency and others won't bother you. Most don't have time. On a visit to the University of California at Berkeley, I witnessed a man in the campus square at noon, performing Tai Chi, by himself, wearing nothing but a G-string.

What time of day would be most beneficial for martial arts training? Research shows that between noon and nine o'clock in the evening is your most advantageous time for punching and kicking. Your reactions, rhythm, strength, and dexterity, are at their peak. Other studies show that your martial arts workout may also feel easier in the evening than in the morning. One way to determine your optimum time to train is to monitor your body temperature. Work out within the three-hour span before, or after your daily temperature high. For most people this occurs at about five o'clock in the evening. Recall whether you stretched, punched, and kicked better when you were cold or warm.

⊃Tips on Training in Public

1. Be inconspicuous.
2. Do not make eye contact with passers-by.
3. Do not block pedestrian or vehicular traffic.
4. Create your own inner world of martial arts.
5. Concentrate on your imaginary opponents.

5.2 Training Solo

As an eleven year old, during the summer, if I had nothing to do I trained at the martial arts studio by myself. Training alone you are masterless. You may not have a particular instructor or style. Whether your goal is to reach the Olympics or improve your self defense, solo training will help.

Imagine training alone for years—practicing punches, kicks, strikes, blocks, footwork, and bag work all by yourself. Doesn't sound like much fun, does it? For most people it is difficult to stay motivated when training alone. But there are benefits. You can concentrate on your training without distraction. You can practice specific techniques that work for your individual body type and temperament. And you can work on weaknesses you might not normally practice in front of others.

The following program is a guide to solo training. It is designed to give you a routine that will keep your skills sharp and, more importantly, keep you motivated to sustain a training regime:

Step 1: Mentally prepare yourself for a rigorous training session. To do this, imagine the "feel" of what it is like after a tremendous training session. Also, "see" yourself as having achieved your martial arts training goals.

Step 2: Allow no interruptions! Take the phone off of the hook and lock the doors. This is your practice time.

Step 3: While you are preparing to begin, if thoughts such as, "I can do this later" or "I don't have time for all of this," enter your mind, then see a big red stop sign forcing these negative thoughts to cease, and remember your goals.

Step 4: Training aids such as a full-length mirror, a radio, etc. are fine. Furthermore, make sure that you have easy access to water.

Step 5: Begin training with abdominals and then jump rope for at least five minutes. Watch yourself in a mirror, and let your thoughts drift to the goals of your training.

Step 6: After warming up with the rope, do some stretching. Be sure to hold each stretch; it will help you to relax as you move to the point of muscle tension. At the same time imagine your muscles as being pliable like rubber bands.

Step 7: Between songs while the radio is playing commercials, practice stances and plyometrics until the next song comes up. When you hear the next song beginning, get ready to perform combinations.

Step 8: Now that you are fully warmed up, it is time to perform full-power combinations on the bag. Tune the radio to a station you really enjoy. Next, as you begin to hear the first song, perform your first combination over and over for the duration of the song. Each song will last approximately three minutes. (Think of the radio as your trainer. If the song goes longer than three minutes, you must have needed the extra practice.)

Step 9: Cool down with some stretching.

5.3 Strength Training

I begin each day with a muscle toning and strength regimen. My strength training program includes lifting weights for forty-five minutes. I train two different body parts at high intensity. On Mondays I work my chest and triceps. On Tuesdays my back, and legs. On Wednesdays my shoulders and biceps. On Thursdays, Fridays, and Saturdays, I repeat the cycle. Total body strength is an asset in martial arts.

There is no better way to contour and streamline your physique than lifting weights. You cannot spot-lose body fat, but you can tone-up and increase the size and strength of your muscles. Increasing the size of your shoulders and upper back creates the illusion of reducing your waistline. Unless you inject illegal supplements, you should not be concerned about being transformed into the Hulk.

Push Ups vs. Weight Training

Countless times I have observed martial arts students attempting to build big muscles by doing hundreds of pushups. Pushups are a terrific warmup, and you can enhance your muscular endurance by doing pushups. But to improve your overall strength, you also need resistance training. Here's why:

When doing pushups, the first phase of your improvement is due to neurological efficiency. You learn to recruit muscles in your chest, shoulders, and triceps. Resistance provided by your body weight while doing pushups is adequate, at first. The second phase of your development is from strengthened connective tissue. Tendons and ligaments in your chest, shoulders, and arms support your newfound muscle.

But to enjoy a third phase of progression, you must add weight training to your regimen. Your muscles are hungry for increased stress. Weight training intensifies the overload on your muscles. More total muscle fibers are required to move the poundage. Your muscles adapt to heavier loads by growing larger and stronger.

You have two basic types of muscle fibers: Type I and Type II. The muscles that sustain your stances are mostly Type I. They are endurance muscles, red, and are considered slow twitch. These muscles are activated repeatedly throughout your workout.

Type I fibers are recruited during pushups and are capable of less force, but can help you perform more repetitions (reps) and last longer than Type II fibers. Pushups are excellent for enhancing Type I slow twitch fiber utilization.

Type I fibers utilize oxygen, which means they are aerobic. They are smaller and contain less glycogen (a type of sugar used as an energy source) than Type II fibers, but their blood-oxygen content is high. They contain capillaries and provide endurance for performing quantities of pushups.

There are two subclasses of Type II fibers; Type II-a and Type II-b. Type II-a intermediate fibers are somewhat oxidative. They use a combination of aerobic and glycogen systems. They are recruited after Type I fibers. Type II-a intermediate fibers are fast twitch with moderate myoglobin content, capillary density, force production and endurance.

Type II-b fibers are non-oxidative (not aerobic). They are strong and provide force, but they fatigue quickly. Type II-b fibers are anaerobic with a high glycogen content and fast twitch rate. They have few capillaries and low endurance but a high power output. Type II-b fibers are required for fast, powerful punches and kicks. To build Type II-b white fast twitch fibers, high intensity weight training is vital.

If you perform twenty pushups, the first several repetitions utilize primarily Type I fibers. Next, Type II-a intermediate fibers assist. To recruit your Type II-b fibers, overload your muscles by increasing the tonnage, i.e. lift weights.

In conclusion, to optimize your program, do pushups and weight training. Pushups provide you with muscular endurance, using primarily Type I red endurance fibers. Train with weights to isolate Type II-b fibers and increase your absolute strength. In addition, high intensity strength training also increases bone mass and bone density.

Free Weights vs. Machines

Lying on your back and bench pressing hundreds of pounds of weight does not necessarily transfer to your martial arts. You could not necessarily push that same amount of weight if it was in human form. In an upright position you would have difficulty counter-balancing the weight. You are only as strong as your ability to stabilize your body.

What this means is that the more similar a training exercise is to your actual martial arts, the more likely it will benefit you. This is known as 'specificity.' It refers to the similarity between a training activity and your martial arts performance. This includes movement patterns, peak force, rate of force development, acceleration, and velocity.

For example, if you are doing a competition form that requires you to land on one leg after a flying spinning hook kick, you would benefit from one-legged step ups, which require you to support your entire body weight on one leg. A normal squat requires both legs balance the weight and therefore may not be as advantageous to improving flying spinning hook kick performance.

Free weights allow muscle contractions similar to your martial arts motions, since movements take place on three planes and are not being guided or restricted as with machine weights. In addition, large muscle mass exercises are more easily accomplished with free weights. Because these exercises require more energy they are more likely to lead to positive changes in body composition.

Training with complex multi-joint exercises using free weights can produce excellent results. Free weights allow movements that are more mechanically similar to those occurring naturally. Considering the evidence that specificity of exercise results in a greater transfer of training effect, free weights should produce an effective training transfer to your martial arts.

Free weights also allow a wide range of incremental weight increases. And although it is commonly believed that machines are safer than free weights, there is no evidence to support this belief. Machines may or may not save time in the gym. The time spent training is largely determined by the length of rest periods between sets.

No studies have indicated that machine training produces better results compared to free weights. For your martial arts training, free weights are your best bet. However, if you have easier access to machine weights, by all means take advantage of them. The use of machine weights will still increase your overall strength and muscle mass.

To conclude this section, here's a cautionary tale. I was doing bench presses in a martial arts studio one day, and could not budge the weight from my chest. I screamed in desperation to my instructor. He shouted back from his office, "I'm on the phone, be with you in a minute." I rolled the bar down my chest to my stomach so that I could sit up and heave it off me. It hurt every inch of the way. From then on, I've had a spotter.

Strength Goals

Lifting weights can increase your strength, flexibility, and muscular endurance. Train with resistance equipment three times each week for an hour. The key to improving your strength and your muscular endurance is high-intensity training. Focus your concentration on a specific muscle group.

For example, to train your chest and triceps, focus on the pectoral muscles in your chest. Concentrate on pushing with the triceps muscles in the back of your arms. Relax the rest of your body so a higher percentage of force is exerted behind the specific muscle groups you are working.

When using weights, attempt to keep your facial muscles relaxed. You can yell if you want, but the parts of your body not doing the lifting should remain relaxed. Imagine a surge of power as the blood enters the working muscle. Explode into each movement with a controlled and yet one-hundred percent energized effort. Move the weight through a full range of motion. Exhale on the exertion. Choose a weight that you can comfortably control. If you are using free weights, be sure to have a spotter. Do not be afraid to call for help if you cannot lift the weight off of your chest.

Individualize your strength program to meet your needs and goals. Take the responsibility to develop your own program. You will find it is easier to adhere to a self-designed training schedule. Prior to each workout, plan the order of your exercises, and the intensity of the training system you have designed. Get psyched up for each workout. Music can be a great motivator. To become energized, think of your martial arts goals and visualize your ideal self. Avoid working out around interruptions such as phones, food, and children. If interrupted, make a note where you stopped.

Do not work out in extreme heat. If it is hot, drink water between sets. If you train in cold weather, do a few calisthenics (i.e. push-ups, crunches, pull-ups) to warm up. Ease in to your workout. Start with some easy repetitions, then gradually increase the intensity. Breathe normally during an exercise; however if you are exerting, exhale during the contraction. Inhale on your short rests between each contraction. Maintain good posture; keep your stomach in; relax your neck; when on a bench, keep your back flat (don't arch). The amount of weight you lift should never dictate your form.

You will see improvement after approximately five weeks. Keep charts to record how you are advancing in each of your muscle groups. Train each muscle group no more than two times per week. Your muscles will adapt to the weight. As you increase the weight and the number of repetitions, you will gain size and strength. For maximum strength gain, do six repetitions. Each repetition should be so intense that you reach exhaustion by the sixth. A mirror is helpful—if you use it for exercise form only! Fixing your hair or checking your smile will not benefit your weight training performance.

Weights Work

Perform one exercise per body part. Work the large muscle groups of the legs, back, and chest first. Stretch each muscle group following each set. Do both high repetition, light weight, and low repetition, heavy weight, to stimulate slow-twitch and fast-twitch muscle fibers. A method to combine heavy and light weight training is to do a "burnout." Start with a weight heavy enough that you can only manage six repetitions. Immediately following your set, remove ten pounds from each side of the bar and do eight repetitions. Continue to remove ten pounds from each side of the bar until you are lifting the bar alone. I was doing a burnout set and a student walked in just as I was struggling on my last set with the bar. He grinned and asked, "How many years have you been lifting?" I replied, "Someday, you too will be able to lift a bar."

In approximately one month, your body will have adapted to your resistance program. To continue to stimulate muscle growth you must add intensity to your workout. You can choose to increase the number of sets, repetitions, or the amount of weight you are lifting. Or you may decrease your rest time between sets. As you lift, keep a log so that you know what you want to adjust. Listen to your body. If your muscles are growing larger, stronger, and more flexible, and you are not gaining additional body fat, you are doing everything right. If your goal is to improve endurance, work your large muscle groups in rapid succession. Do not dawdle between exercises. If you rest too long you may lose "the pump," and decide to quit for the day. I lock the doors to the gym until my students finish their workout.

Follow The Experts: Periodization

Ask yourself four questions: What are your strength training goals? How do you plan to achieve them? How much time are you willing to spend training? And what type of strength training equipment is available to you?

There are several stages in your strength training periodization development. Your adaptation stage allows you to establish a training base from which to build upon. At first, your intensity is low to moderate, with high volume. The strength stage requires a moderate volume and high intensity. The number of repetitions decreases from the adaptation stage. But the amount of weight you are lifting increases. A muscular endurance stage is a combination of high strength development and adequate endurance. This stage uses high volume and low to moderate intensities. Strength is converted to endurance by increasing the duration of your exercise. In the next stage, strength is converted to power by increasing movement speed.

The power stage is for advanced weight trainers. The purpose of this stage is to recruit fast twitch muscle fibers. This stage employs low volume and high to very high intensities. Most exercises are performed at near-maximum weight. Other exercises are executed with low weight but a high speed of movement. The maintenance stage is used during your off season from martial arts competition. Cross-training is encouraged, to maintain your conditioning.

Divide your training year into periods, each with a specific physiological purpose. Build strength in stages, much the same as constructing a house. When a period is completed, evaluate your progress. The strength benefits accrued are sustained through each succeeding period. Then, other muscle groups are developed. Continue setting and achieving new strength goals until you are satisfied with your performance.

A series of training sessions called microcycles make up your training program. Microcycles are your daily and weekly training sessions. Microcycles include variations in exercise volume, intensity, and selection. Your training plan is termed a mesocycle. It may last from a month to a few months. For optimum results, a mesocycle should proceed without interruption. Usually a mesocycle begins with several exercises and plenty of repetitions. Remain consistent on your mesocycle regimen. Be careful not to skip training sessions. And more importantly, do not overtrain. Your mesocycle is consummated with a high intensity peaking phase, followed by a lower intensity recovery break.

Although there are no set rules for mesocycle programs, generally progression continues for three weeks. The fourth week is the end of your mesocycle. This last week is lower intensity, and is used to recover. The next mesocycle begins after your recovery period.

A macrocycle is the sum of your mesocycles. It may range anywhere from a few months to a few years. Your macrocycle requires alternating various intensities. Your goal is to peak at specific times of the year. Depending on your metabolic requirements, certain training protocols may be employed more than once, while others may never be used.

Plan a series of mesocycles to accomplish your goals. Evaluate each mesocycle. Make decisions about your progression. Add intensity, variety, and cross-training to each mesocycle when necessary. Include a mesocycle of recovery or active rest. A standard practice is to lower your effort after three weeks of continuous workouts. This reduces your risk of overtraining or injury.

After active rest, your next mesocycle will begin at a slightly lower intensity. Then, increase your intensity according to the design of your next mesocycle. Figure out the frequency, intensity, and duration necessary to achieve your targets in each phase of your progression. The number of phases and amount of time spent in each phase will depend on your fitness level and your specific goals.

Evaluate yourself regularly to monitor your progress. Determine if your program needs any alterations or fine tuning. Changing up your training program decreases your potential for overuse injuries. And you avoid overtraining. Periodization promotes an optimal response to the training stimulus. It encourages consistent physical improvements, avoiding your tendency to plateau. You stay fresh and motivated. This improves your adherence and enjoyment.

Train Smart, Not Hard

Some peoples' standard of training is using information provided by the most muscular person in the gym. "Arnold (Schwarzenegger) looked like Arnold long before he began weight training" according to Ellington Darden, Ph.D. Just because Arnold does it, doesn't make it right.

Training systems have changed. Years ago, bodybuilders performed partial repetitions to pump up their muscles. They did not work their muscles through a full range of motion. Short movements increased strength only at the angle that the muscle was working and only provided a thirty to forty percent strength increase.

Some bodybuilders spend incredible amounts of time in the gym. Research demonstrates however, that an hour and a half is all an individual needs to stimulate muscle during a training session.

Gym rats may use a dozen different exercises to work the biceps at different angles to change its shape. You cannot change the shape of a muscle. Electromyographical studies have indicated that if you could only do one exercise to stimulate all three biceps flexors, straight bar curls are your best bet.

Along those lines, some bodybuilders suggest doing endless sets of hand twisting movements when performing the military press. Again electromyography showed that a simple military press performed in front of the neck stimulates all three heads of the deltoid. And, in-front-of-the-neck presses are safer than performing behind-the-neck presses.

The same goes for lat. pull downs. For safety reasons as well as following the line of pull of the muscle, draw the bar down in front of your neck. A case study revealed that a woman performing behind-the-neck lat. pull downs ruptured a disk in her cervical spine, causing paralysis.

Many bodybuilders attempt to train their posterior deltoid (rear shoulder) by doing bent over flies. The problem with this exercise is that it innervates the rhomboids (upper back) and trapezius (the muscles beside your neck) with little stimulation to the rear deltoid. To work the back of your shoulders, grab some light dumbbells and lie prone (face down) on a bench. Lift the weights so they are parallel to your shoulders. From this position, turn your pinky toward the ceiling and perform a three inch movement flexing your posterior deltoid on each repetition.

You may notice that most exercisers raise their hips when they perform prone leg curls. The reason they unconsciously do this is that raising their hips pre-stretches their hamstrings so they can get more force into their contraction. The only problem with this technique is that it may aggravate disk problems in the lower back. Another way to get more out of your hamstrings when you perform the leg curl is to keep your feet relaxed through the full range of motion. If you point your toes toward your knees (dorsi flex) you inadvertently use your calf muscles (gastrocnemius) to aid you in lifting the resistance. Allow your feet to relax or point (plantar flex) your toes and your gastrocnemius will not help your hamstring hoist the weight.

Women are notorious for having problems with their vastus medialis (the ligaments and muscles on the inside of the knee). Sometimes these tissues are not strong enough causing their knees to bow inward at the slightest pressure. The patella (knee cap) may sit off to the side creating painful bone to bone contact. Performing leg extensions and leg curls may strengthen her quadriceps and hamstrings to improve patella tracking.

When you perform triceps extensions you probably try not to use momentum during the exercise. There are three heads of the triceps. When you use a slight bit of momentum to raise the weight a tad higher, you innervate the part of your triceps just below your shoulder. Try it. You may discover a muscle you never trained before.

You probably would prefer to optimize your time in the gym. Develop specific goals and sculpt your body to meet your needs. Countless times I have walked into gyms and watched bodybuilders attempting to work their obliques (waist muscles) by holding a broomstick on their shoulders and twisting from side to side. Your obliques are innervated only when you flex both forward and sideways simultaneously. Furthermore, some bodybuilders make a distinction between training their upper and lower abs. As mentioned in chapter two, the rectus abdominis is a long straplike muscle that extends from the ribs to the pubis. You cannot work your upper and lower rectus abdominis independently because it is a single muscle.

5.4 Using Dumbbells

When training with dumbbells, it is not as important to have a partner with you to "spot" you as when you are using barbells. However, having a partner can be beneficial. While you concentrate on lifting, your partner can keep an eye on your form to make sure you move through full range of motion, maintain good posture, and don't hold your breath. A partner can also encourage you to finish those last two or three reps that are making your muscles burn and shake.

As you go through the following program, decide for yourself the number of repetitions of each exercise, as well as the amount of weight. To train your muscular endurance, perform more reps at a lighter weight. To train strength, increase the weight and lower the number of repetitions.

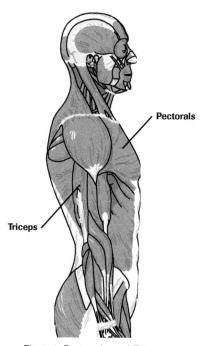

Fig 5-1. Pectorals and Triceps

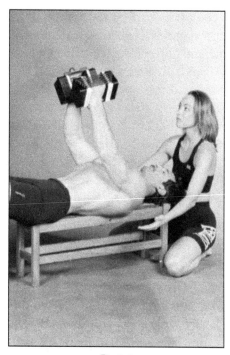

Fig 5-2

Lying Five

Bench flies for the pectorals and triceps (Figure 5-1): Lie on your back on a bench, grasp the dumbbells in an overhand grip (Figure 5-2), and extend your arms from your chest level upwards (Figure 5-3). Have enough weight to provide tension so you can keep the dumbbells moving smoothly and evenly. Keep your elbows slightly bent through the full range of motion. Feel your chest and triceps working. Keep the back of your head, buttocks, and lower back in contact with the bench.

Pullovers for the latissimus dorsi and pectorals (Figure 5-4): Lie on your back and grip the dumbbell with both hands. Extend the dumbbell back over your head as the bar dumbbell provides resistance (Figure 5-5). Then flex it back in the opposite direction (Figure 5-6). Feel a stretch in your upper back and chest.

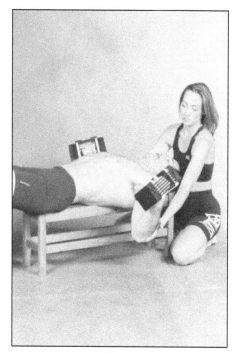

Fig 5-3

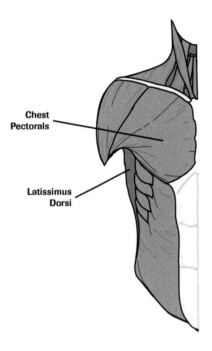

Chest
Pectorals

Latissimus
Dorsi

Fig 5-4. Latissimus Dorsi and Chest

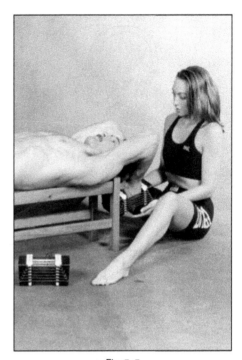

Fig 5-5

Posterior raises for the rhomboids and rear deltoids (Figure 5-7): Lie on your stomach and grip one dumbbell in each hand (Figure 5-8). Raise the dumbbells from the floor until they are a few inches above parallel (Figure 5-9). Then slowly lower them back towards the floor. Keep your elbows bent for the duration of the exercise.

Lateral raises for the lateral deltoids (Figure 5-10): Lie on your side holding one dumbbell with your top hand (Figure 5-11). Raise the dumbbell from the floor up to a vertical position (Figure 5-12) and then slowly lower it back towards the floor. Repeat with your other arm.

Triceps extensions: Lie on your back holding one dumbbell in your right hand (Figure 5-13). Extend the dumbbell into a vertical position (Figure 5-14) and then slowly lower it back towards your left shoulder. Repeat with your left hand.

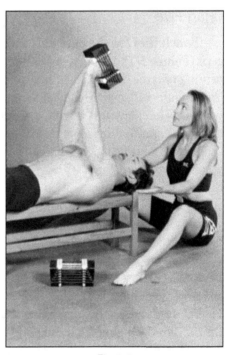

Fig 5-6

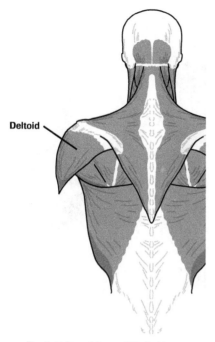

Fig 5-7. Rear View of Deltoid

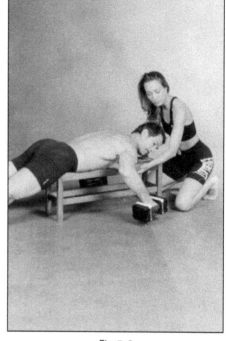

Fig 5-8

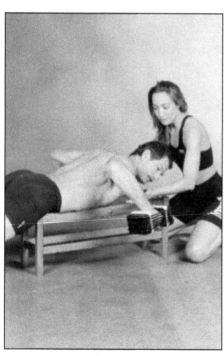

Fig 5-9

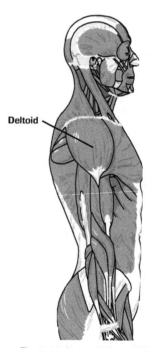

Fig 5-10. Lateral View of Deltoid

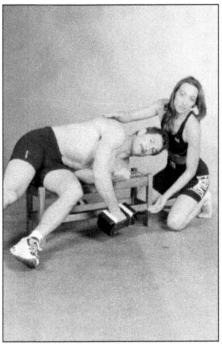

Fig 5-11

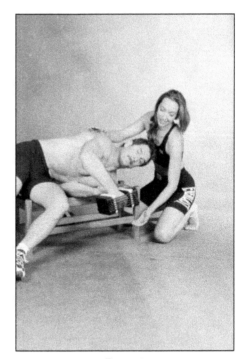

Fig 5-12

Sit for Six

Triceps kickbacks: While on your hands and knees grasp a dumbbell with one hand with your elbow at a 90 degree angle (Figure 5-15). Extend your arm straight back until your elbow is locked (Figure 5-16). Hold for one second then return to the ninety degree angle. Repeat with your other arm.

Single-handed lat. work for the latissimus dorsi: Grab the dumbbell with one hand while the same knee is braced on a bench. Extend the arm as far down as you can toward your side and feel a pulling sensation in your lats (Figure 5-17). Then lift the dumbbell to your hip as the resistance presses down (Figure 5-18). Reverse hands and make sure to move through a full range of motion.

Shoulder press for the deltoids and triceps: Sit on a bench with good posture, holding the dumbbells on the back of your shoulders (Figure 5-19). With the dumbbells

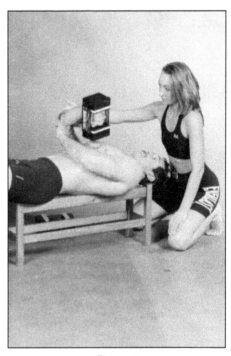

Fig 5-13

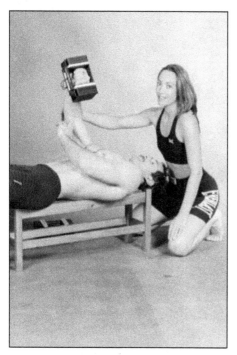

Fig 5-14

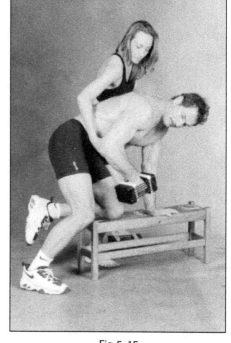

Fig 5-15

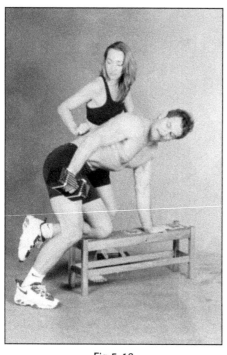

Fig 5-16

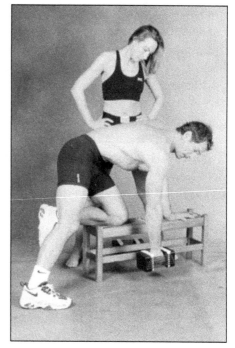

Fig 5-17

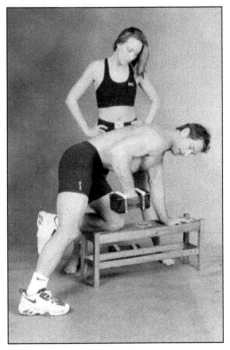

Fig 5-18

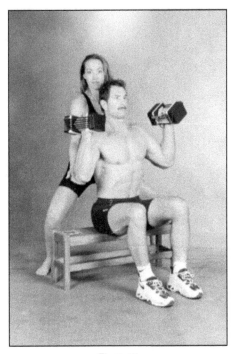

Fig 5-19

in an overhand grip, press them toward the ceiling as the resistance presses down (Figure 5-20). Keep your torso and head in a straight line with your chest out. Push with equal pressure from each arm upward to full extension. As you lower the dumbbells slowly toward your shoulders, keep constant tension.

One-armed curls for the biceps (Figure 5-21): Grip the dumbbell with your right hand as the left hand supports the right arm to isolate the tension in the biceps (Figure 5-22). Lift and lower the bar through the full range of motion while moving the bar at a semi-circular angle with the elbow joint as the fulcrum (Figure 5-23).

More triceps work: Sit on the bench holding one dumbbell behind your neck (Figure 5-24). Extend the bar upward as the resistance presses downward until your arm is straight (Figure 5-25). Feel the tension in the back of your arm. Let the resistance provide pressure in both directions. Switch hands and repeat.

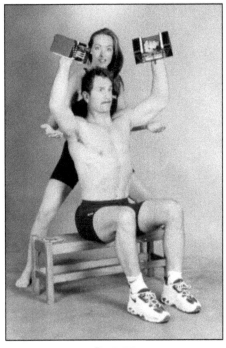

Fig 5-20

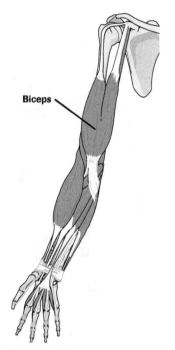

Fig 5-21. Biceps

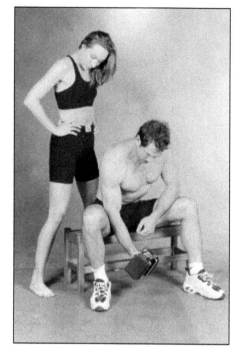

Fig 5-22

Shoulder flies for the deltoids: Sit with a dumbbell in each hand (Figure 5-26). Lead with your elbows as you lift them parallel to the floor, working the lateral aspect of your shoulders. Slowly raise your arms upward (Figure 5-27). The weight should provide tension in both directions.

Stand for Seven

Bent over row lat. work for the latissimus dorsi and back: While bending from the waist, keep your head up and bend your knees and grasp the dumbbells in an overhand grip with your hands a little more than shoulder width apart (Figure 5-28). Keep your lower back slightly arched and pull the dumbbells up toward your chest, keeping your elbows close against your body (Figure 5-29). Maintain a neutral spine, and lower the dumbbells in a straight line back towards the floor (Figure 5-30).

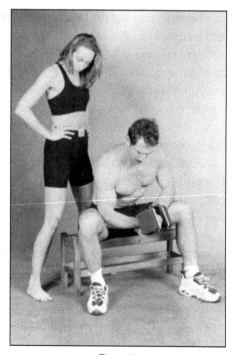

Fig 5-23

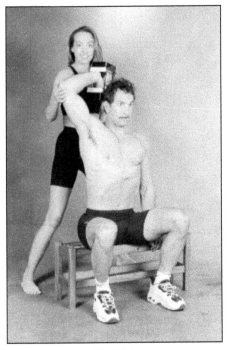

Fig 5-24

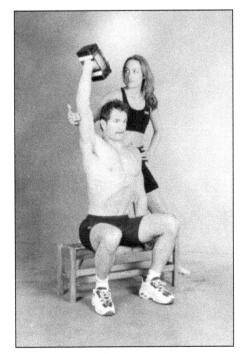

Fig 5-25

Reverse curl for the brachioradialis and biceps: Grip the dumbbells at thigh level with an overhand grip, hands a little less than shoulder width apart (Figure 5-31). Bring the arms up from the waist to shoulder level until your biceps touch your forearms (Figure 5-32). Lower the weights back down to your thighs using your elbows as the fulcrum.

Arm curl for the biceps brachii: Grasp the dumbbells in an underhand grip, palms up, arms close to your sides. Allow the dumbbells to rest against your thighs (Figure 5-33). Pull the dumbbells toward your chin in a semicircle until your forearms touch your biceps (Figure 5-34). Keep your wrists locked. Lower the dumbbells on the same path you lifted them. Move the bars up and down slowly through the full range of motion.

Anterior deltoid for the shoulders: Grab the dumbbells with your hands about shoulder width apart and your palms facing downward in front of your thighs (Figure

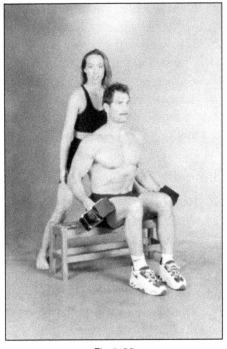

Fig 5-26

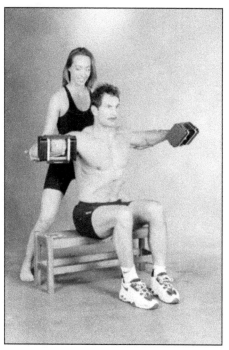

Fig 5-27

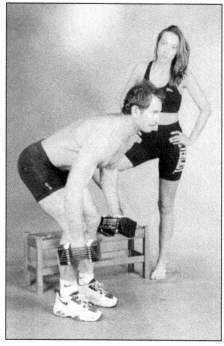

Fig 5-28

5-35). Keep your knees and elbows slightly bent, and slowly raise the dumbbells toward your head. Pause when your arms are parallel to the floor (Figure 5-36), and then slowly lower them back towards your thighs.

Trapezius training for the upper shoulders: Grab the dumbbells with your palms facing downward, your hands together and your arms extended so that the dumbbells rest against your thighs (Figure 5-37). Bring the dumbbells up toward your chin while leading with the elbows so that they flare out to the sides up to your ears (Figure 5-38). Keep constant tension throughout the full range of motion as the dumbbells remain close to your body. At the top of the movement pause and flex your trapezius muscles. This exercise if contraindicated if you have shoulder pain.

More trapezius training: Grab the dumbbells with an overhand grip, palms down, your hands shoulder width apart and your arms down to your sides (Figure 5-39).

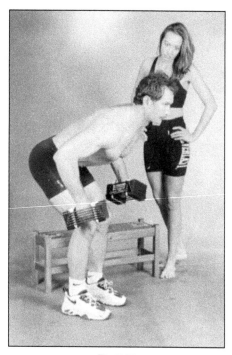

Fig 5-29

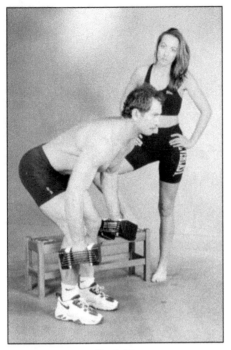

Fig 5-30

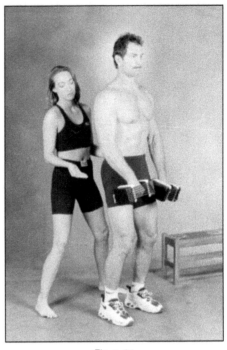

Fig 5-31

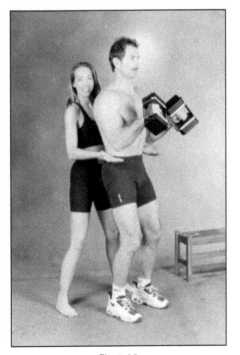

Fig 5-32

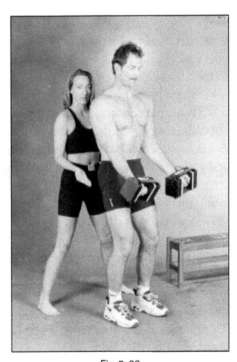

Fig 5-33

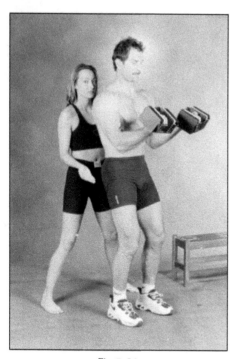

Fig 5-34

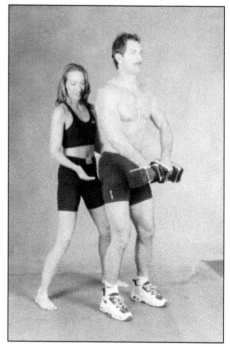

Fig 5-35

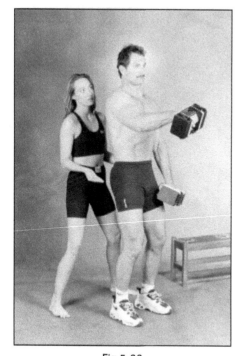

Fig 5-36

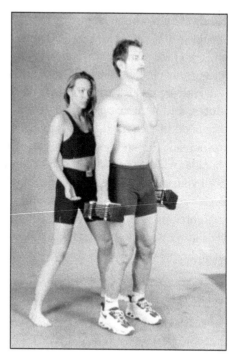

Fig 5-37

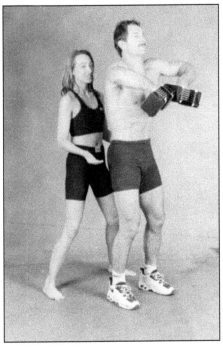

Fig 5-38

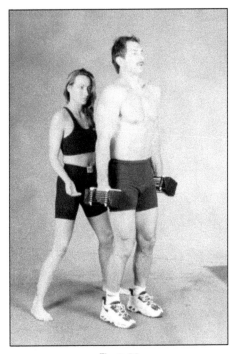

Fig 5-39

Keep your elbows straight as you drop your shoulders down as far as you can (Figure 5-40) and then raise them up to your ears with the weight providing resistance in both directions.

Half-squats for the quadriceps, glutes, and hamstrings: Stand with a dumbbell in each hand, arms extended down to your side (Figure 5-41). With your feet shoulder width apart, slowly bend your knees until your upper thighs reach a forty-five degree angle (Figure 5-42). Pause and straighten up again. Keep your head up and your lower back slightly arched. Your knees should remain over your toes.

⟳Tips on Resistance Training

1. Choose a weight you can comfortably work with for ten repetitions.
2. Perform each exercise through the full range of motion.
3. Exhale on the exertion phase of each movement.

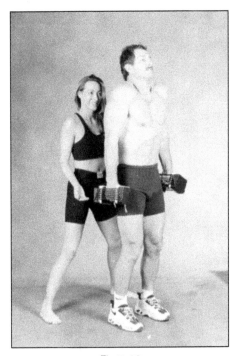

Fig 5-40

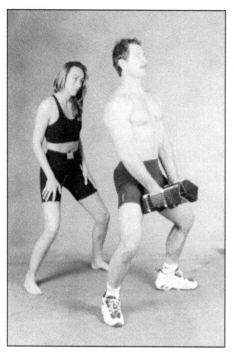

Fig 5-41

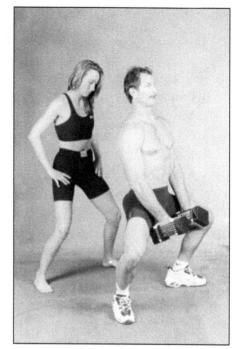

Fig 5-42

4. Relax muscle groups that are not involved in the lift.

5. Perform each exercise with perfect posture.

6. Move slowly, never jerking or bouncing the weight.

7. Stretch after each set.

5.5 Mind Over Muscle

You may feel a burning sensation in your muscles as you increase your intensity. Soon you will anticipate the burn. The burn, and fatigue in the muscles, are a signal that you are approaching muscular failure. If you occasionally work your muscles to failure, you will see tremendous strength gains.

Reaching muscular failure is difficult because you must endure some discomfort. One way to do this is to focus your attention on the muscle group you are working. Or you may disassociate yourself from the pain. I use a combination of both techniques. During my first few repetitions, I disassociate by thinking about my upcoming set. However, during my last few repetitions, I focus on my muscles growing stronger and more powerful. Changing your mind about discomfort can change your body. Increasing strength is your measure for success.

How to Delight In Discomfort

Do not use the following pain control technique to mask injury. See a physician for an acute injury or for pain that lasts more than a week. Follow the steps below to endure the fatigue and discomfort of a workout.

1. Fatigue exists in your mind.
2. You can beat fatigue and discomfort.
3. Go with it. Pushing yourself through discomfort will lead you to your goal.
4. Increase your intensity. Expect an increase in discomfort.
5. An increase in "the burn" is a signal you are closing in on your goal.
6. You are objective about the burn and fatigue. Observe it. Enjoy it.

Spend time daydreaming about your workout. Close your eyes prior to each set. Take thirty seconds to see, feel, and experience each repetition. Do no permit negative thoughts. If you are in the middle of an exercise and you think "I'm tired, I'm not going to finish," then immediately change your thought to, "STOP, I was tired, but I'll push it out, complete my training, and feel great." You can use self-hypnosis, positive imaging, positive self-statements, relaxation, positive suggestion, prayer, anything but anabolic steroids, to keep you in the proper frame of mind.

If you reach a plateau in strength, change your training routine. Modify the sequence of your exercises, do different exercises, increase your intensity, upgrade your diet, sleep more, decrease the frequency of your workouts, or paint a fifty-five on your forty-five pound plates.

Most of us would be satisfied to gain lean muscle, lose body fat, and maintain flexibility and cardiovascular endurance. A combination of weight training, aerobics, and proper eating is the solution. To build lean muscle, use a high-intensity resistance program. I have seen enthusiastic bodybuilders attempting to build muscle on the stairmaster, exercise bicycle, versa-climber, and treadmill. These machines are designed to enhance cardiovascular endurance, not increase size and strength.

Upon reaching your strength and size goals, less intensity is required to maintain your muscularity. Studies have shown that weight training one day a week can stimulate your muscle fibers to remain toned. However, if you miss more than two months of training, than consider yourself starting from square one. Therefore, once you start a program, do not quit. If you do quit, do not quit altogether. It is easier to stay in shape than it is to get there.

○Tips on Minding Your Muscles

1. Imagine yourself lifting the bar off the rack. Feel the cold steel in your hands.
2. Feel the pressure of the weight as it drops slowly and controlled to your chest.
3. As the bar arrives at your chest, see and feel yourself extend the bar upward to full extension.
4. Hear the clang of the bar as you replace it on the rack.

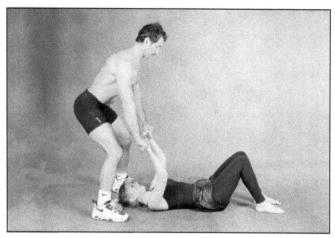

Fig 5-43

5.6 If You Don't Have Weights

If you do not have access to resistance equipment, do push-ups, crunches, and pull-ups. My muscle-strengthening program began when I was thirteen years old. I was a television addict. On commercials I would do push-ups. Soon I could do sixty push-ups in each one-minute commercial.

You can also use the bar synergism routine I have developed. All you need is a bar and a friend. The friend could be your spouse, child, or training partner. Instead of loading your bar with weights, use your partner to provide the resistance. One of you pushes, the other pulls. In a half-hour you can systematically train every muscle in your body.

Bar Exercises

Lat. work for the latissimus dorsi and back: While bending at the waist keep your lower back slightly arched, grasp the bar in an overhand grip with your hands a little more than shoulder width apart (Figure 5-43). Pull the bar up toward your chest (Figure 5-44). Your partner should be lying with his/her back on the floor to provide resistance in a downward direction as you pull up. Keep your knees slightly bent. Maintain a neutral spine throughout the entire exercise to prevent injury.

Back strengthener for the rhomboid muscle (Figure 5-45): Sit facing each other. Place the bottoms of your feet together and bend your knees slightly. Both you and your partner grab the bar (Figure 5-46). One of you should begin leaning toward the floor at a forty-five degree angle as the other person gives constant resistance through the full range of motion. Alternate pushing and pulling with your partner (Figure 5-47).

Bench press for the pectorals and triceps: Lie on your back and grasp the bar in an overhand grip (Figure 5-48). Extend your arms from your chest level upwards (Figure 5-49). Your partner presses down with enough tension so you can keep the bar moving smoothly. Keep your elbows in. Feel your chest and triceps working.

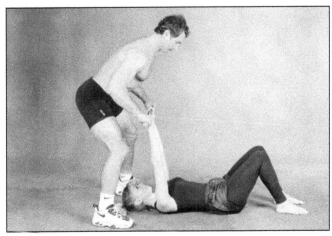

Fig 5-44

Arm curl for the biceps: Stand facing your partner. Grasp the bar in an underhand grip, arms close to your sides (Figure 5-50). Pull the bar toward your chin as you partner pushes downward (Figure 5-51). Keep your wrist locked. Move the bar up and down slowly, through the full range of motion.

Shoulder press for the deltoids and triceps: Sit on a bench with the bar resting on the back of your shoulders (Figure 5-52). Grasp the bar in an overhand grip and press the bar toward the ceiling as you partner presses down (Figure 5-53). Push with equal pressure from each arm upward to full extension. As you lower the bar toward your shoulders have your partner keep constant tension.

Reverse curl for the brachioradialis and biceps: Grip the bar at waist level with an overhand grip, hands a little less than shoulder width apart (Figure 5-54); bring your arms up from your waist (Figure 5-55).

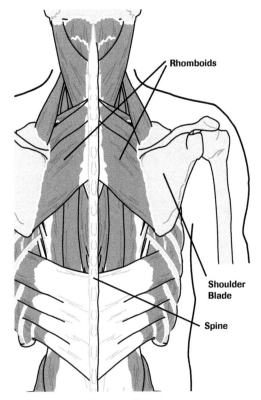

Fig 5-45. Rhomboids

Triceps reverse grip pull-downs: Use an overhand grip with your hands close together (Figure 5-56). Keep your elbows tucked into your body as you press the bar toward your knees (Figure 5-57). Your partner should apply pressure in a upward direction until your arms are extended, then in a downward direction until your arms are bent at ninety degrees.

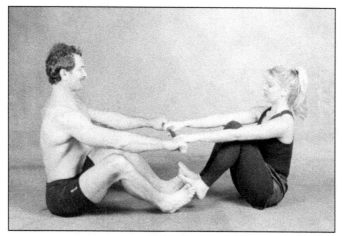

Fig 5-46

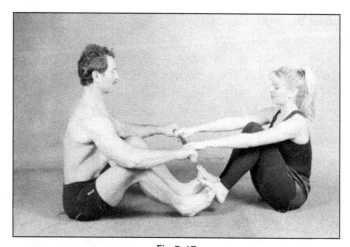

Fig 5-47

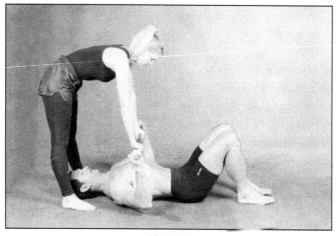

Fig 5-48

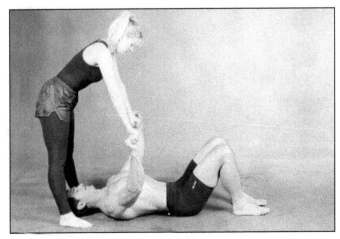

Fig 5-49

Single handed lat. work for the latissimus dorsi: Grab the bar with one hand while the same knee is braced on a bench. Extend the arm as far down as you can toward your side and feel a pulling sensation in your lats (Figure 5-58). Then lift the bar to your hip as your partner presses down (Figure 5-59). Reverse hands as your partner applies equal pressure in both directions through the full range of motion.

Pullovers for the latissimus dorsi and chest: Lie on your back and grip the bar with both hands, less than shoulder width apart (Figure 5-60). Extend the bar back over your head as your partner applies resistance (Figure 5-61). Then flex it back in the opposite direction. Feel a stretch in your upper back and chest.

Biceps and triceps work: Lie on your back, grab the bar in the center with your hands actually touching. Place the bar one

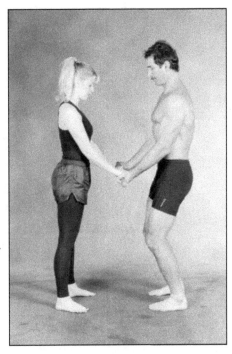

Fig 5-50

inch from your chest (Figure 5-62). Extend the bar upward with your partner's resistance (Figure 5-63). Pull back down toward your chest with resistance. Reverse your grip and perform another set. As you extend you will be working your triceps; as you flex you will work your biceps.

Heavy back work for the back and biceps: Grab the bar with a close grip and bend over at your waist with a flat back. Extend your arms toward the ground with your partner's body weight as resistance. Flex your arms back up to your chest and feel a

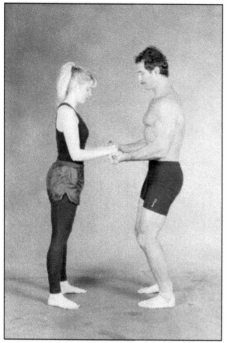

Fig 5-51

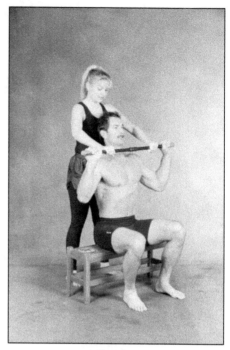

Fig 5-52

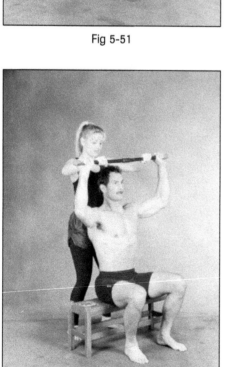

Fig 5-53

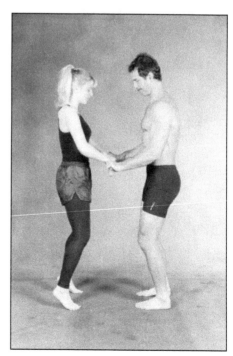

Fig 5-54

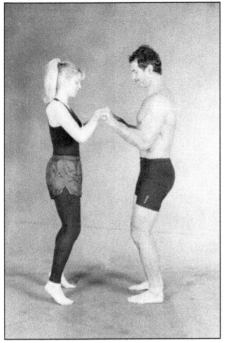

Fig 5-55

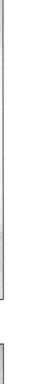

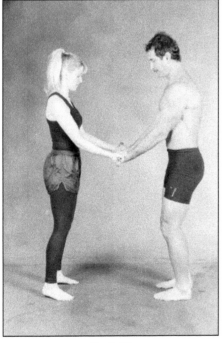

Fig 5-56

Fig 5-57

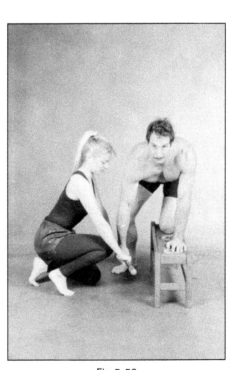

Fig 5-58

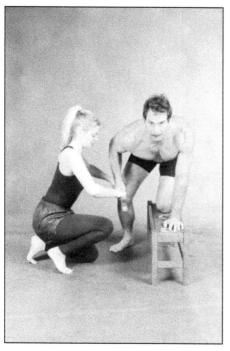

Fig 5-59

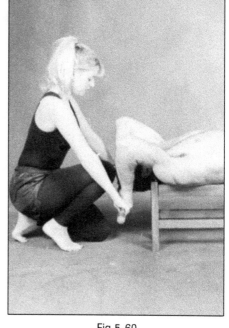

Fig 5-60

tremendous pull on the back and biceps (Figure 5-64). You should feel both a stretch and tension in the lats.

Wide-grip pull-ups for the latissimus dorsi and forearms: Put the bar between two props and grab the outer handles (Figure 5-65); perform as many behind-the-neck pull-ups as possible (Figure 5-66). Lead with your elbows through a full range of motion.

Close-grip pull-ups for the latissimus dorsi and forearms: Put the bar between two props and grab it (Figure 5-67). Pull yourself up to chest level.

Close grip bench for the triceps and chest: Lie on your back with the bar on your chest. Grasp the bar with an overhand grip (Figure 5-68). With your hands close together, press up toward the ceiling to full extension (Figure 5-69). Your partner should provide tension in both directions.

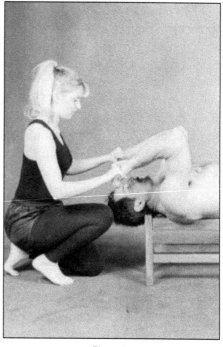

Fig 5-61

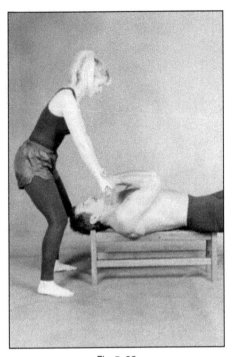

Fig 5-62

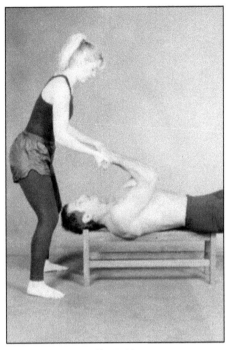

Fig 5-63

More biceps work for the biceps and forearms: Lie on your back. Grasp the bar in an underhand grip with your hands together. Extend the bar above your chest (Figure 5-70). Pull the bar toward your forehead as your partner provides tension in both directions (Figure 5-71).

Frontal deltoid for the shoulders: Grab the bar with your hands about shoulder width apart and your palms facing downward. Extend your arms so the bar is down by your knees (Figure 5-72). Slowly raise the bar toward your head without bending your elbows (Figure 5-73). Your partner should be standing in front of you to provide upward resistance.

Trapezius training for the upper shoulders: Grab the bar with your palms facing downward, your hands together and your arms extended (Figure 5-74). Bring the bar up toward your chin while leading with

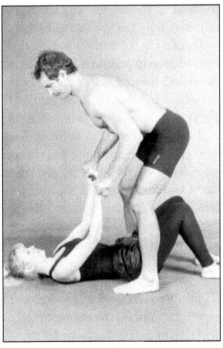

Fig 5-64

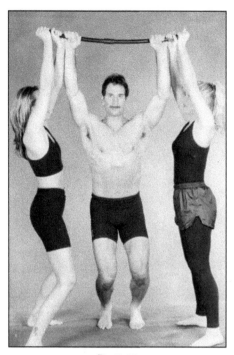

Fig 5-65

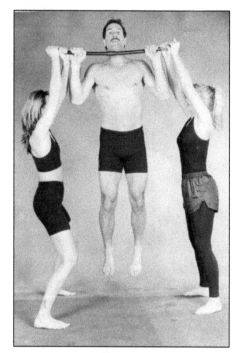

Fig 5-66

the elbows. Your partner should provide
resistance on the way up (Figure 5-75). Flex
your trapezius. This exercise is contraindicated if you have shoulder pain.

Shoulder shrugs for the trapezius:
Grab the bar with an overhand grip, your
hands shoulder width apart and your arms
down to your sides (Figure 5-76). Keep your
elbows straight as you pull your shoulders up
to your ears with your partner providing
resistance in both directions (Figure 5-77).

Shoulder flies for the deltoids: Sit
with your partner behind you. With your
arms out the sides, lead with your elbows as
your partner applies pressure to the back of
your wrists (Figure 5-78). Slowly raise your
arms upward (Figure 5-79). Let your partner
provide tension in both directions.

**Mini pull ups for the lats and fore-
arms:** Sit with your legs extended in front of
you. Grab the bar with both hands in an over-

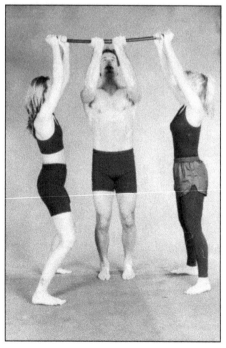

Fig 5-67

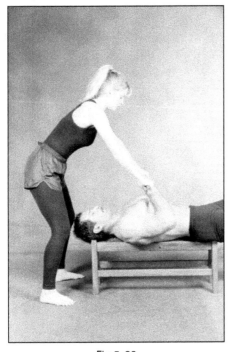

Fig 5-68

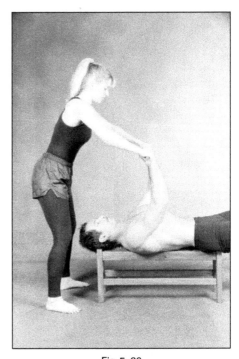

Fig 5-69

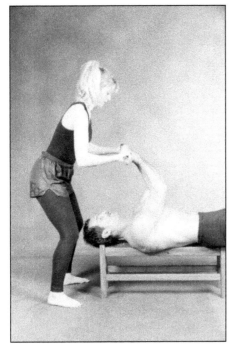

Fig 5-70

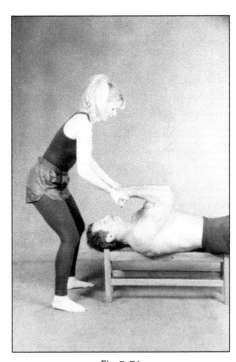

Fig 5-71

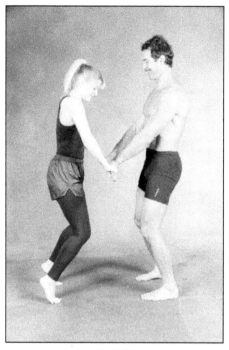

Fig 5-72

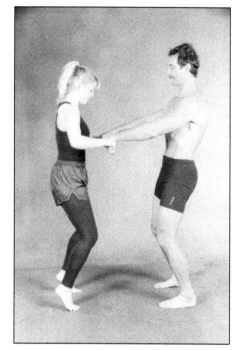

Fig 5-73

hand grip (Figure 5-80). Let your partner hold the bar in a braced position as you perform as many pull-ups as you can (Figure 5-81).

Neck work: With the bar and pad on your forehead, let your partner push as you push with your neck (Figure 5-82). Flex and extend slowly and comfortably in both directions. Use the same procedure for the sides of your neck (Figure 5-83).

⮌Bar Synergism Tips

1. Seconds prior to performing a set, visualize the groove you will take the bar through.
2. Attempt to isolate the muscle group you are working.
3. Use the palm-heel of your hand if your grip is weaker than the muscle group you are working.
4. Use a specific sequence of bar-synergism exercises, working the large muscle groups first.

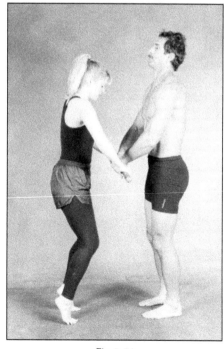

Fig 5-74

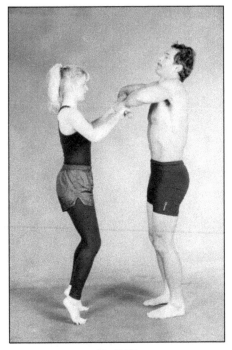

Fig 5-75

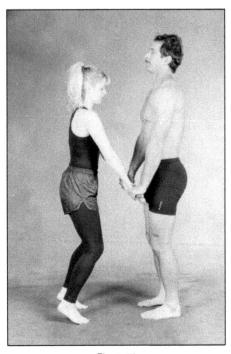

Fig 5-76

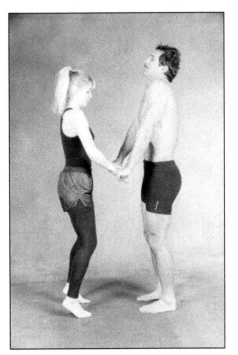

Fig 5-77

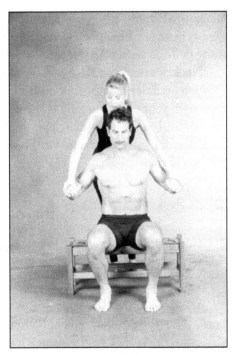

Fig 5-78

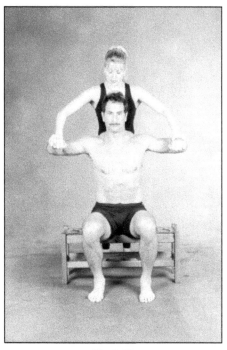

Fig 5-79

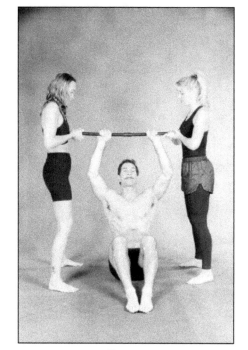

Fig 5-80

5. If you are not strong enough to give your partner adequate resistance, have your partner work one arm at a time.

6. When you are helping your partner perform an exercise, maintain equal resistance with each hand.

7. Perform each movement through a full range of motion.

8. Resist your partner on both the concentric (going up) and eccentric (coming down) phase of the contraction.

9. Be sensitive to your partner's movement. Apply enough pressure to require your partner to work slowly through ten repetitions.

10. Maintain correct posture. Keep your stomach in, your neck relaxed, and your lower back slightly arched.

11. Warm up before an intense workout and cool down afterward.

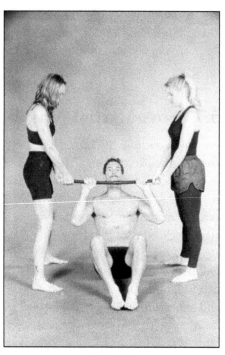

Fig 5-81

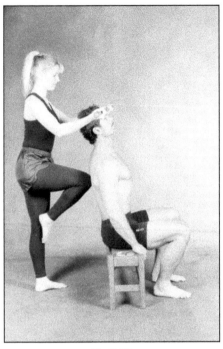

Fig 5-82

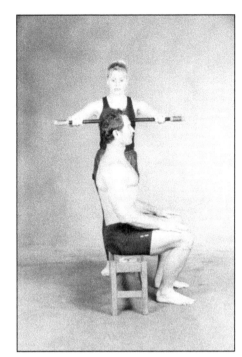

Fig 5-83

12. Remain relaxed except for the muscle group you are working.
13. When spotting for your partner, apply slow, smooth, and balanced pressure. Avoid one arm pulling harder than the other.

5.7 Cross-Martial Arts Training

Cross-training has kept me in the best shape of my life. I can work out six hours a day without overtraining. The key to my regimen is alternating high-impact and low-impact exercises with different strength, cardiovascular, and flexibility programs. Four days a week I lift weights, ride the Stairmaster, do aerobics and plyometrics, play tennis, practice martial arts, and ride a rowing machine. The other three days I circuit weight train, cycle outdoors, and stretch.

Any sport that improves your flexibility, strength, endurance, and concentration will help you master your art. Your sedentary peers may complain about joint stiffness and weight problems while you achieve higher levels of strength, flexibility, and endurance. Other beneficial effects of cross-training include: increased reaction time, toned muscles, enhanced alertness, decreased blood pressure, and a lower resting heart rate. In addition, a variety of psychological benefits such as increased self-esteem and self-discipline may enable you to live a happier, healthier life.

Martial arts, tennis, weight training, cycling, concentration training, prayer, and all of the peripherals that accompany each of these activities is my path to master my art. I wake up training and fall asleep planning my next day's program.

Sports can get us in shape or out of balance. You can gain tremendous endurance from running marathons but not have the strength to carry a suitcase. A weight lifter can hoist a car but be injury-prone because of one-dimensional training. Martial arts offer a well-rounded workout. The training can improve your performance in many sports, and sometimes provides a needed break so you can attack work or studies with renewed vigor. Not only is martial arts a catharsis, but research shows that focus may be transferred from your training to the work place or to other disciplines.

A martial artist must hit fast and hard at a very small target, or pull a kick less than one inch from the opponent's face, or lock a training partner's joint without tearing ligaments or breaking bones. These skills require a combination of both power and grace, performed with speed, balance, and control, in an atmosphere of strict discipline. These skills may also help you hit a baseball or make a sale. In return, other sports may benefit your martial arts. For example a baseball pitch and the knife hand strike have similar arm motions.

A personal example is tennis (Figure 5-84). Tennis took my time in the mornings, and I punched and kicked at night. Transfer effects include enhanced footwork, improved speed of strikes and tennis volleys, and weight transfer of tennis strokes and strikes.

Some martial arts instructors emphasize running to improve endurance, but I think cycling is better (Figure 5-85). Unlike running, cycling does not tighten hamstring muscles. Furthermore, cycling is low-impact, allowing feet, ankles, knees, and hips a needed rest from the bone-jarring pounding of martial arts. Outdoor cycling is more beneficial than stationary riding because of the hills, breeze, and scenery. You can ride with a buddy or alone. If you cycle solo, you can mentally rehearse your forms or sparring, but keep your eyes on the road. Wear a helmet and be careful of dogs and cars.

Cross-training water-based workouts is another way to improve your endurance and take the stress off your joints. Head for the nearest pool and try this: sit on the edge of a pool and flutter kick your legs back and forth in the water until you feel warmed up. Then step down into the shallow end and perform your stretching exercises. The water helps keep you relaxed. Next, practice all of your basic kicks, blocks, and punches using the water as resistance. Do your forms in slow motion. Maintain perfect form. Finish up with a couple laps of easy swimming.

Cross-training is not just physical. Seemingly disparate pursuits can be intertwined. Master your art in every experience you encounter. Call it cross-training for life. While driving to work switch off the radio and focus your concentration. Transform a boring job into a body language or social studies experiment. At home do your chores mindfully. Acknowledge the interconnectedness of all you do.

⊃Cross-Martial Arts Training Tips

1. Sports like racquetball, ping-pong, basketball, and tennis can enhance your hand-eye coordination, reaction time, and footwork.

2. Long-distance jogging, cycling, and swimming can give your overall stamina a boost.

3. Short sprints can optimize your ability to perform quick, powerful movements.

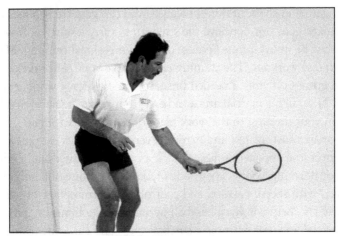

Fig 5-84

4. Gymnastics, soccer, and skating can contribute a tremendous amount of leg strength, flexibility, and coordination.

5. You may work out alone, with a partner, or with a group.

6. You can progressively improve your techniques as you continue to train.

7. You may reduce stress in your life.

8. Cross-training burns calories which can help you lose weight, strengthen your arms and legs, and increase your muscle tone.

Cross-Brain Training

I was a teenager when I first enrolled in transcendental meditation (T.M.). The first day of class we were required to bring a handkerchief, an apple, and thirty-five dollars. The instructor taught us to recite a mantra, a word theoretically designed for each of us. We were instructed to repeat this mantra silently for twenty minutes. If any distracting thoughts or sounds disturbed us we were told simply to let them go in one ear and out the other. When we thought the twenty-minute time period was up, we should open one eye and glance at our watch. More often than not, I would awaken from a deep sleep with my chin nestled on my chest. However, over time I was able to quiet my mind enough to relax and experience an inner sense of peace.

You don't have to perform sitting meditation to enjoy the benefits of a calm quiet mind. Basic training, combinations, forms, and sparring are a sample of the myriad of activities that open capillaries and stimulate pleasure centers in the brain. Researchers at the Dallas Aerobics Center have demonstrated stress reduction and longevity benefits when exercising large muscle groups in a relaxed cadence for twenty minutes. Cross-training exercises can become a form of meditation.

If you say you don't have time to fit in cross-training or meditation, try this: set your alarm thirty minutes early. Start your day with twenty minutes of invigorating forms or a leisurely mantric respite. Personalize your program to meet your needs. Whether you jump rope or meditate, relaxation, concentration and repetition will

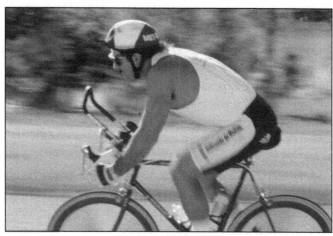

Fig 5-85

decrease anxiety and promote vigor. The long-term benefits are worth that extra half hour of sleep. And if you're concerned about being tired, go to bed a half hour earlier to make up for it.

Below are some cross-training exercises you can do for a mind and body workout. You can do many of these exercises first thing in the morning to start your day.

Jump Rope: Stand on the middle of your rope and raise the handles to your armpits. Turn the rope easily at a relaxed cadence. Relax the muscles in your shoulders and arms. Bounce low, without jolt or impact. Breathe comfortably. If you are panting or wheezing slow down. Look straight ahead. Free your mind and let thoughts travel effortlessly.

Indoor Cycling: Adjust the seat so your knees are slightly bent when you extend your leg downward. Relax your upper body and turn the pedals in perfect circles. Spin smooth and steady. If your leg muscles burn, lessen the resistance. Listen to music and let your mind wander. Continue with the beat and pedal briskly without overexertion.

Pump Iron: Combine resistance training with aerobics by circuit training. Do ten repetitions at a weight that lets you comfortably perform all ten repetitions. Move from one exercise to another as quickly as possible. Exhale on the exertion of each repetition and consciously flex each muscle you are working. Enjoy the pump, without strain.

Metaphysical Golf: Save the cart-fee and golf becomes worthwhile. Step lively between holes. Lug your own bag. Gerald Fletcher, M.D., wrote that golf improves agility, mental acuity, focus, and friendships. If you add relaxation, fresh air, and walking, the benefits can be enormous. An average nine-hole course is two miles, and eighteen holes is a four-mile workout.

Non-Competitive Partner Activities: Throwing or kicking a ball back and forth, smacking a paddle ball, racquetball, ping-pong ball, or tennis ball are rhythmic if you stroke balls cooperatively. Swat serves on the run. While waiting to return, stay light on your feet. Your opponent is your accomplice. Your ego never assaults the court. Speed-walk to gather balls between rallies.

Mind/Body Basketball: A basketball pick-up game can be mind altering. Shuffle and shadow-box between power jams. Your feet never stop. Get open or cover a man.

Listen to music. Music adds rhythm to the game. Get started and keep going.

In-Line Skating: Every Saturday I do aerobic baby-sitting. I take my children for a relaxing roller-blade/stroller ride to the playground. My kids enjoy the breeze while I maintain a constant rhythmic pace with my arms and legs. Develop a side-to-side movement. Swing your arms for balance and speed.

Step-Ups: Upon arriving at the playground, I pull my running shoes from the stroller and practice step-ups on a miniature balance beam while my kids play on the equipment. You can do step-ups on almost any playground apparatus. Try step-ups on a four inch bench. Watch your feet as you put your right foot up, then your left foot, then your right foot down, and your left foot. Keep your feet close to the bench. Place your entire foot on the bench. Step off on the ball of your foot and then roll to your heel. Feel the muscles in your legs contract and relax. Progress gradually to prevent injury. After a while you won't be bothered about your pace. Stepping will come as naturally as walking and your mind can wander.

Stair Climbing: An even safer method of step-ups is the stair climbing machine. Researchers at California State University at Northridge demonstrated that runners had several dropouts while the stair climbers had no injuries or dropouts. Stair climbing is considered low impact because your feet never leave the machine. There is no strain on ligaments or joints, and you control the intensity. The hum of the machine is your mantra.

Rowing: If you don't have a canoe, indoor rowing is a low impact total body workout. It exercises your hips, abdominals, arms, trunk, legs, and shoulders. The repetitive motion is as natural as swaying back and forth in a rocker. Once you gain coordination, your mind is free to ponder the universe.

Fitness Walking: Researchers at Brown University found that the government could save money on down-time and health care if they paid people to walk. Walking is easy, and you can do it anywhere. You can walk with a friend or go solo. Swing your arms for an extra workout, or focus on your breathing as you enjoy the fresh air.

Backpacking And Hiking: Backpacking is an easy escape. A one hour hike over uneven terrain is comparable to a three mile walk, not to mention the energy expenditure of carrying a pack. Backpacking is a natural—just remember to take a compass.

Cross-Country Skiing: Cross-country skiing trains both your lower and upper body. The large amount of muscle mass involved makes cross-country skiing intense, but it places little pressure on joints. Moving smooth and steady increases velocity. You control your acceleration. And the scenery cannot be beat.

Swimming: Back problems or knee pain may prevent you from walking or jogging. A non-impact, aerobic answer is swimming. Feel the texture of the water and savor the solitude. Find your steady state and enjoy.

Outdoor Cycling: Cycling is rehabilitative. Breathe deeply from your diaphragm instead of puffing from your chest. Pedal as fast as you can without pain or strain. Spin fast rpm's rather than pushing big gears. Change the position of your hands often and stand up regularly. Feel the breeze and hear your tires spin.

Flexing And Stretching: Flex your triceps before you stretch your biceps, which forces your biceps to relax automatically. Then alternate flexing biceps and stretching triceps. Flex and stretch every antagonist muscle group in the body. Pay attention to the feel.

Stretching And Breathing: Begin at your neck and stretch every muscle sequentially until you reach your toes. A slow, continuous stretch is desired. Exhale as you move into each position. Hold for twenty seconds. Slowly stretch to the limits of joint motion, until you feel tension in your muscles. Then relax. Go for comfort. Stretch at home or at work.

Instead of coffee, let your twenty minute morning routine be your pep pill. Spend the next eighteen hours feeling great. While others are drinking cokes and scarfing donuts, reflect back to your twenty minute routine. Break it down into a manageable mini-strategy to impart instant energy. Grab a minute-mantra break, take a deep breath in the car, or tap your toes to simulate action. If you can steal five minutes, zone out or stretch out or shadow box. Or focus on your heartbeat during a boring meeting. Stretch and then flex muscles at your desk or calmly walk to the fountain. Remember, you don't have to be in your uniform or on your meditation cushion to train.

⤷Tips on Cross-Brain Training

1. Choose a cross-training activity you are comfortable with.
2. Your activity should be an enjoyable adjunct to your martial arts training, not an additional source of stress.
3. Be sure your activity is relaxing and non-competitive.
4. Use your activity to promote peace of mind.

5.8 Team Training

My first full-contact fight took place in Plano, Texas. My opponent (also his first full-contact fight) and I were both extremely nervous. Ed Daniels, my trainer, was a legend in martial arts. I followed every bit of his advice, but I should have declined his decision to spread heat balm all over my body to "warm me up." I was on fire. I attacked so vigorously I forgot the fight was scheduled for five rounds. Fortunately so did my opponent. Rounds two through five turned into a waltz, neither of us having the energy to raise a hand or foot. Rather then pace ourselves we expended all of our energy in one shot.

Martial arts is considered an individual sport, and you may feel quite alone in the ring or on the floor. However, you might be selected or choose to compete for a team (Figure 5-86). This happens when you fight for your school, state, or nation. It takes a lot of team chemistry to win an international title. If a single member of a team dissents, the rest of the team may fall. The chemistry between team members plays a criti-

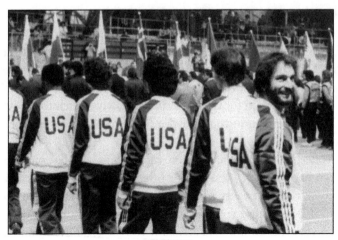

Fig 5-86

cal role in whether or not you win. When team members are on the same page, and the team works well together, they can accomplish almost anything. But most competitors know little about team work. They know when things are going well, but they don't know why.

Team members may be serious or relaxed. Some may be goal oriented and others fun loving. The more contrast in personalities the better balanced the team may be. Regardless of personality style, each team member must feel comfortable communicating with the rest of the team. When a team member is in the ring, find out whether he or she prefers shouts of support or advice. For example a teammate may say "great kick," or "you're open to the body." When your teammate returns to the corner, whether he or she is winning or losing, be sure your body language is encouraging. There is nothing more depressing than a corner man with slumped, defeated shoulders although the bout is only half over. Treat your teammate the way you would want to be treated in the same situation.

Teammates may be friends for life. Each member should try to understand each others needs. Some competitors fight best when they remain standing, tense and focused between rounds. Others sit deep into their chairs and relax. Some are talkative when they are nervous. Others just want to be alone. Try to understand what each martial artist needs to perform at his or her best (Figure 5-87).

➲Team Training Tips

1. If you know your teammate has a weakness, turn it into a strength. Don't wait until it is too late.

2. Don't try to change too much too soon.

3. Whenever you change a movement be prepared for a few uncomfortable moments when your old habit no longer works and the new technique has not fully blossomed.

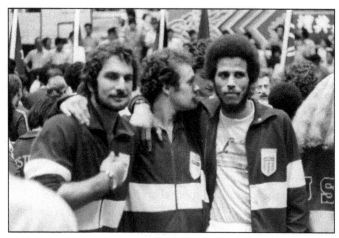

Fig 5-87

4. Keep your teammates pumped up between rounds even when they are tired or discouraged.

5. Plan your sparring strategy prior to each round.

6. Follow the same rituals before beginning every round.

7. Be acutely tuned into your teammates' matches.

8. Project a confident image regardless of the score.

5.9 Nutrition for Peak Performance

Fighting in tournaments taught me a lot about nutrition. The morning of a contest I woke up with my buddies for a fast-food breakfast of scrambled eggs, sausage, bacon, toast, juice, and milk. Then we rushed to registration only to learn we wouldn't be fighting until about noon. We watched the forms competition and by two o'clock in the afternoon we realized we would not compete until five P.M. Our blood sugar and energy levels dropped, and some of us were so burned out from pre-contest anxiety, dehydration, and low blood sugar that we considered sleeping instead of competing. Our nerves were frayed and we lost our appetites. By the time we entered the ring, adrenaline was our fuel source. Our bodies consumed muscle for energy.

If I had a tournament tomorrow, I would wake up to a breakfast of pancakes, scrambled egg-whites, toast, juice and milk. I would eat a piece of fruit or an energy bar every two hours to stabilize my blood sugar. For variety I may have a bowl of cereal and skim milk for breakfast, followed by a carbohydrate drink taken at two hour intervals throughout the day. When it was fight time, I'd be ready.

The last snack before your competition should be something that will fuel you up but not stick to your stomach. Lots of fighters use carbo drinks and energy bars. They stoke up on bars and drinks before their bout, drink them between rounds to help sustain their power, and enjoy them afterward to replace depleted glucose stores and lost nutrients. Whether competing in a day-long tournament, getting in a hard workout, or simply sparring with your buddy, energy bars and drinks might improve your performance. Most contain easily-digested carbohydrates, and they fit conveniently into your gym bag.

My eating habits during the week weren't any better than my tournament habits. To save money I ate one all-you-can-eat meal each evening. My metabolism slowed and I gained body fat. Furthermore, I was lethargic, and my martial arts training suffered. Similar to a sumo wrestler, my body efficiently stored fat.

Eating no breakfast, a skimpy lunch, and a large dinner is the most common eating pattern of people in America, and a most efficient method of gaining body fat. Skipping breakfast or lunch leaves you famished at supper, resulting in overeating and a sluggish metabolism. Those who skip breakfast more than make up for those calories later in the day. They carry more body fat too. When more than a few hours pass between meals, blood sugar drops, energy drops, and fatigue sets in.

Some claim that proper nutrition is simply eating three square meals a day from the four food groups. It's not that simple, but it is easy. Eating correctly may not be the magic bullet, but if you don't eat right, you have less chance to reach your goals.

Your Training Table

If you took a month's worth of food to a martial arts camp, you wouldn't eat it all the first week. Likewise, rather than consuming three large meals in a day, spread your calories into six daily meals. Eating six times a day, you never get too hungry. Your mini-meals should contain nutritious foods you may normally forget to eat, especially fruits and vegetables. In ancient times pigging out on a large feast was a luxury. Cave dwellers spent most of their time grazing on leaves, roots, and berries throughout the day. Six small feedings a day will provide increased energy for your training.

Moving from three to six meals a day also helps lower your low density lipoprotein (LDL) cholesterol, according to McGrath and Gibney in the 1994 *European Journal of Clinical Nutrition.* Excess LDL cholesterol clogs your arteries, blocking blood flow to the heart.

A report in the *New England Journal Of Medicine* revealed the need to eat several meals each day, rather than just two or three. Those who grazed on seventeen meals found that their food was absorbed more efficiently and the nutrients were utilized more effectively. (Seventeen! I'm only suggesting you eat six). In addition their metabolic rates increased and they lost body fat. Another study suggests you should eat a variety of different protein-amino acid combinations, complex carbohydrates, and mono-unsaturated fats. It is also important to vary the number of calories you eat on a daily basis so your body doesn't adapt and lower its metabolism.

Another study showed that eating six meals a day lowers insulin levels, decreasing cravings and subsequent binges. After three weeks of eating six quality meals a day, greasy foods and rich desserts are no longer to die for. You will desire what your body needs, not what some television commercial fools you into believing. My meals include a combination of protein such as chicken breasts, turkey breasts, fish, yogurt, cottage cheese, egg whites, or lean red meat with carbohydrates including fruits, vegetables, cereals, grains, or breads.

Eating frequently is an effective plan for any martial artist. Consume three meals and three mini-meals each day and add extra carbohydrates for your post-workout meals. Your body muscles twice as many grams of carbohydrates twice as fast if you consume them within thirty minutes of your workout. This window of opportunity is the best time to refuel muscle and liver glycogen stores.

When you increase the frequency, intensity, or duration of your martial arts training, add calories to each meal. Your six small meals should include a serving of protein and two servings of a carbohydrate at each sitting. The body can store only limited amounts of excess carbohydrates as glycogen, mostly in the liver and in muscle, while fat can be distributed all through the body. Carbohydrate storage is carefully regulated. Fat storage is not. A study at the University of Leeds showed that breakfast eaters who ate more fat were hungry soon after their meal more than those who bulked up on the same amount of carbohydrate calories. A martial artist attempting to lose body fat might consume:

Breakfast: Five scrambled egg whites, oatmeal, and toast.

Mini-meal: Yogurt and an apple.

Lunch: Turkey sandwich with fruit and vegetables.

Mini-meal: Rice cakes, non-fat cheese, carrots, and celery.

Dinner: Baked chicken, baked potato, and green beans.

Mini-meal: Fiber cereal, lowfat milk.

Eating for energy is essential to martial arts success. Individualize your eating to your workouts, but basic dietary truths apply for all athletes. Steer clear of too much fat and sugar and develop a taste for lean proteins, fibrous vegetables, and starchy carbohydrates. Develop an ongoing trial-and-error eating plan.

Research suggests endurance athletes require more protein than other athletes; therefore, martial artists may find it beneficial to increase their intake of both protein and carbohydrates.

Snacks

If you miss a meal, have a snack. Be careful that your snack does not trigger a binge. Many of us are addicted to high fat, high sugar foods that have little nutrition. Baked chicken, tuna, brown rice, and egg whites may not compare to ice cream, hot dogs, and cotton candy, but your tastes can be modified and your habits altered. A quick trip through your local supermarket's produce section will reveal a host of ready-to-eat fruits and vegetables, as well as other nutritious snacks that make it convenient to eat right.

Fat-free snacks are better for you than fatty ones, but fat-free is not a license to gorge. (Although I'm probably not the only one who has eaten a box of fat-free cookies in a single sitting.) An Oreo has two grams of fat per cookie while Snackwell's Devil's Food Cookie Cake is fat-free. Eating fat-free cookies is better than fat-laden ones, but that's still a lot of calories and sugar. Remember, "fat-free" does not equal "calorie free."

Eat to Lose

Have you ever gone on a diet and discovered your discipline melted when you opened the freezer? You had the best intentions, but nothing on earth could loosen your grip on those ice cream bars. Diets don't work because when you cut calories you crave the very same foods you are attempting to avoid. And it probably was not due to lack of willpower that you could not stick to your diet. Temporary diets never keep the fat off. You may lose weight on the scale but you also lose water and muscle. When you resume normal eating, you gain more fat because your metabolism has slowed.

The answer to long term weight management lies in making wise food choices; and eating frequently throughout the day. Food comes in many varieties. Breads, cereals, fruits, vegetables, dairy, and meats are necessary for survival, but overindulgence in these very same foods causes obesity, heart disease, and diabetes. Therefore discipline, along with the knowledge of when, how much, and what foods to eat are your ingredients to successful eating.

Make wise food choices a lifelong habit. Training in martial arts requires patience and self control; so does staying on a proper eating plan. If you can spend three hours in the training hall, you can find three hours a week to shape up your eating.

Eating correctly and martial arts are skills. Both must be learned and practiced before becoming habit. It takes about three weeks to become accustomed to your new eating program and then it is easy. There are two rules you must follow:

1. Never go hungry. Eat every few hours to stabilize your blood sugar.
2. Have your healthy foods available so you aren't tempted by morsels that are not on your eating plan.

Sabotage is just around each corner. Fatigue can weaken your resolve. Heavy training or working eighty hour weeks can diminish your ability to make proper eating choices. Pace yourself. Schedule your meals in advance so you will not succumb to fast food temptation. Bring food with you. Buy a cooler and carry fruits and vegetables with you. Initially it was difficult getting in meals between breakfast and lunch, and between lunch and dinner. Now I enjoy pre-cut vegetables and chicken or non-fat yogurt while my colleagues are wolfing down soft drinks and chips.

Stress can cause undereating, which eventually leads to a binge. Others eat compulsively when they are anxious. And you can bet their food choices are full of fat. If you need to de-stress, instead of grabbing a brownie, practice one of the relaxation techniques in this book, or think about your martial arts training.

Trying too hard to be perfect is self-defeating. Obsessing about a goal makes it impossible to reach. If you say, "I can't ever eat ice cream again," all you will think about is ice cream. Instead focus on your victory over ice cream and go on.

Food can act as a drug. Eating large quantities of carbohydrates at lunch increases serotonin in the bloodstream, leading to mid-afternoon lethargy. But you can fuel your body according to your needs. Regulate types and quantities of proteins and carbohydrates to allow you to feel any way you wish. A consistent pattern of eating can stabilize blood sugar and keep you energetic. You can even alter your moods with your new style of eating. Frequent feedings stave off hunger and allow you to "feel" in control.

We blame the "fat gene," low self esteem, or a sedentary job on being overweight, but we make choices to be fit or fat. You can be a slave to food and feel deprived, or triumphantly decline a second dessert. Just say no to a hot dog and yes to a baked potato. Give yourself a chance to eat healthy. It tastes better when you feel good.

You can watch television or throw some kicks. You can stand in front of the refrigerator or do bag work. Most humans take the easiest path. But not you. Make the right choice. Soon the right decision will become a habit. It's okay to watch television and eat, but view an informative program and consume calories to fuel your muscles for martial arts.

Progress Not Perfection

In a recent study, elementary school students were allowed to choose from a variety of fruits, vegetables, meats, cakes, and ice cream. At first most chose desserts, but within two weeks they switched to fruits and vegetables. Sooner or later, your body lets you know what it needs. A study reported in the May, 1994 issue of the *American Journal of Clinical Nutrition* showed that subjects who ate less fat and more carbohydrates were happier and kept the weight off more effectively than those who simply counted total calories.

In the past, if a cake found its way into my house, I surreptitiously cut thin bite-sized pieces until the entire cake vanished. A half gallon of ice cream would magically disappear from the carton, one shovelful at a time. Nutritionist Keith Klein recommends that if you sneak a piece of cake, don't blow it by consuming the whole cake. If you have a flat tire, would you slash the remaining three tires? Keith advises us to make better bad choices. Instead of chowing down on a carton of ice cream, savor a serving of non-fat frozen yogurt. Rather than blowing it on a pepperoni pizza, create a cheeseless vegetable pizza. Now I occasionally allow myself a treat, and my body-fat is lower than when I pretended to be strict.

Water

Approximately seventy percent of your body is water. Muscles are three quarters water. Blood is eighty-two percent water. Your brain is seventy-six percent water. And your lungs are ninety percent water. Water is needed as a coolant, to digest and absorb food, transport nutrients, build and rebuild cells, lubricate joints and cushion organs and tissues, remove waste products, and enhance circulation. Water is cholesterol free, fat-free, low sodium, calorie free, and one hundred percent natural.

Martial artists don't give water the respect it deserves. True, it does not provide energy, and it is not an anti-oxidant, but water is involved in just about every process in the human body. During the first few hours of water deprivation, blood volume decreases limiting the transportation of nutrients to and from muscles. Losing as little as two percent water hurts performance.

Eight glasses of water a day are enough for couch potatoes, but not for martial artists. Sedentary people lose about twelve ounces of water each day from breathing, and another twenty-four ounces from light perspiration. But many are chronically dehydrated. In

Asia, following each training session my gi was saturated with sweat. Martial artists need about one milliliter of water per calorie expended. That means if you burn two thousand calories, you need an additional two liters (two quarts or eight cups) of water.

Another way to calculate your water requirements is to weigh yourself before and after a workout. For every pound you lose, drink sixteen ounces of water. Drink extra water before your training or event. Four hours before your performance, start drinking eight ounces of water every fifteen minutes.

Your thirst mechanism may malfunction during intense martial arts training, so don't rely on it. If your body fluids are low your brain signals you to drink. But this occurs after you are somewhat dehydrated. In the heat of battle or training, martial artists forget to drink. Extremely active competitors should drink to satisfy their thirst, and then drink some more.

As a white belt overseas, it was my job to provide water. I carried the pitcher outside and filled it with water that was so cloudy and warm that I didn't drink it. Instead, at the conclusion of each class, I ran to the village store and guzzled a large soda. Bad idea. Now I prime the pump by sipping fluids every half hour. I carry a water bottle with me to the training hall for refreshment and to keep me sharp.

Water may not be as glamorous or well advertised as other drinks, but it is essential for life and for good training. If you drink enough water to support your training, the blood-sludgy effects of dehydration will be transformed into super-hydrated peak performance.

Other Fluids

If you are training or competing for more than two hours, research has demonstrated that carbohydrate sports drinks and juices can enhance your martial arts performance. A variety of sports drinks are on the market. Make sure your drink has equal amounts of potassium and sodium (about fifty milligrams in an eight ounce serving). And enjoy the taste (you will drink it if you like it).

Other drinks that fit into your martial arts program may include skim milk (whole milk is fifty percent fat and two percent milk gets thirty-six percent of its calories from fat), limited coffee, and limited tea. Juices are ninety-five percent water, and oranges ninety percent. Also soups, grapes, and yogurt are mostly water. Coffee and tea are ninety-nine percent water, but the caffeine produces a moderate diuretic effect. Of course, clear clean water is always a great choice. Drink enough fluids so that your urine is clear and copious and you feel a need to relieve yourself approximately every two hours.

Energy Bars and Sports Drinks

Energy bars are no better than a banana, fig bar, or cup of yogurt for providing energy for workouts and performance, but they are more convenient. Years ago, eating before exercise was forbidden. Now we understand that eating prior to, and during competition can improve stamina and performance. Up until now, water and sports drinks have cornered the market on pre-fueling for performance, but bars can also boost your energy before and during training and competition.

Your hunger and thirst mechanism may malfunction during intense exercise. Body weight may drop a few pounds before you feel thirsty. I prime the pump by sipping fluids or nibbling energy bars. Carry a bottle filled with water or your favorite energy drink, or rip into a sports bar of your choice.

Bars provide between 150 and 325 calories, with most of the energy coming from carbohydrates (maltodextrins, glucose polymers, oat bran) and simple sugars (corn syrup, fructose, dextrin, and fruit juice.) Some are fat-free and others are loaded with protein. These nutrients fuel your muscles and brain so you can perform your best. Martial artists who forget to eat before training plod through their punches and kicks, lacking energy and enthusiasm.

Try to consume between two hundred and four hundred calories before training and performance. Experiment to find which bars are easily digested. The price of a bar may or may not be worth the convenience of easy storage and accessibility—bars aren't crushed as easily as a banana. Eat a well-balanced diet consisting of real food, but when it comes to quick and convenient pre-performance energy try a bar.

Sports bars and drinks have various functions. Some provide simple sugar for quick energy. Others contain complex carbohydrates and protein for energy, growth, and repair. A few, comprised of thirty percent fat, tout the notion that to lose fat you must ingest fat. And the latest craze is one hundred calorie, disposable packets of instant syrup appropriately termed "GU." For the sake of space, we will discuss the two largest genres of bars.

The "PowerBar" type products contain approximately 250 calories from simple and complex carbohydrates, with a modicum of protein. Many contain high fructose corn syrup and fructose. These products are used for quick energy. "Gatorade" type sports drinks fit this category because of their energy contribution and provision of sodium and potassium.

If you are exercising in excess of two hours, research has demonstrated that carbohydrate drinks, juices, and bars can enhance your performance. Sometimes sports bars and drinks are too sugary. Simply dilute the drinks with water or eat half of a bar and save the other half for later. Look for sports drinks with between ten and twenty grams of carbohydrates per eight ounce serving (more carbohydrates than that decreases fluid absorption into the intestines). Make sure your drink has equal amounts of potassium and sodium (about fifty milligrams in an eight ounce serving). And enjoy the taste (you will drink it if you like it). Quick-energy bars and drinks may contain refined sugar, a syrup derived from fruit, rice, or corn. Beware. Some claim to contain minuscule amounts of "added nutrients."

Another division of bars and drinks are designated as engineered foods. They contain quality protein for muscle growth and repair, with slow release carbohydrates for energy. Recent research suggests the Recommended Daily Allowance (RDA) of protein (0.8 grams per kilogram of body weight), may be too low for active individuals. Peter Lemon Ph.D., renowned for his work on muscle metabolism at Kent State University, encourages endurance and strength athletes to consume one gram of protein per pound of body weight on a daily basis. He advocates athletes eat several small protein portions through the day rather than consuming large quantities at a single sitting. And consuming carbohydrate/protein following a workout refuels muscle glycogen stores.

Because engineered bars and drinks are quick and convenient, they have become America's healthy version of fast-food mini-meals. They range between 250 and 310 calories with about forty grams of protein, thirty grams of carbohydrate, and less than two grams of fat. Many of these engineered foods are packed with vitamins and minerals. They are delicious on-the-road refreshment and are a great quick fix.

However, engineered bars and drinks are not short-cuts to perfect nutrition. They do not replace food. There is no magic elixir. Bars and drinks will come and go, but well-balanced meals are here to stay. And beware of expensive products that promise too much.

Supplements

My five year old son told me that when he takes his multi-vitamin he can feel his muscles grow. He's not the only one who believes in placebos. Supplements are a multi-billion dollar industry. You can purchase anything from herbs to shark cartilage to ginseng. It's hard to resist products that promise increased energy, weight loss, or muscle gain, "for a low, low price." But do they work?

Some doctors contend we get all the vitamins, minerals, and amino acids we need from our food. However, surveys show that Americans consume less than two thirds of the recommended allowance of vitamins and minerals. Fast foods, dieting, and poor eating habits are major contributors to poor nutrition. You should strive for a more healthful diet because of your need for extra energy, and only food provides energy. Without food, vitamins and minerals cannot be absorbed efficiently.

Women martial artists may benefit from a calcium supplement, especially if they don't consume dairy products. Iron may be required to offset their monthly menstrual cycles. Teenagers need extra food and supplements to ensure proper growth and to meet their high energy output. Older athletes could use vitamin B12 and a multi-vitamin mineral supplement to make up for lack of appetite or poor nutritional habits. Vegetarians who eat no meat or dairy need supplements including vitamin D, B12, and riboflavin.

Choose supplements that have at least twenty of the vitamins and minerals shown to be essential for optimum health. Among these, beta-carotene, vitamin C, and vitamin E are antioxidants that have been shown to combat free radicals. Free radicals attack organs, making them susceptible to cancer. Antioxidants destroy the free radicals but are consumed in the process. The more you train, the more free radicals attack your system. Therefore, you need extra antioxidants. Below is a list of vitamins the American Medical Association deems necessary for health, along with the minimum requirements:

Vitamin A .... 250 IU
Vitamin D .... 400 IU
Vitamin E .... 6 IU
Thiamin .... 1 mg

Riboflavin .... 1 mg
Niacin .... 10 mg
Vitamin B6 .... 1.5 mg
Folic Acid .... 100 mcg
Vitamin B12 .... 3 mg
Vitamin C .... 50 mg

⮑Nutrition Tips

1. Under-eating or under-sleeping can lead to over-training.
2. Schedule meals in advance.
3. Become sensitive to your energy needs.
4. Do not skip meals.
5. Eat the right kind of foods.
6. Treat yourself to a "forbidden food" once a week.
7. Eat your high calorie foods in the morning.
8. Eating speeds up your metabolism.
9. Craving sugar may mean that you are not eating enough protein and carbohydrates throughout the day.
10. Take control of your cravings by fueling your body every few hours.
11. Special order low-fat at restaurants. Use tomato, broth, and wine-based sauces instead of high-fat gravy, cream, and cheese sauces.
12. Buy large quantities of brown rice, oatmeal, tuna, potatoes, and large bags of chicken breast, vegetables, and cereal when they are on sale.
13. Make small changes: Skim milk instead of regular, jelly on toast instead of butter, mustard on sandwiches instead of mayonnaise, water or juice instead of soda, non-fat frozen desserts instead of high-fat frozen yogurt, non-fat salad dressing, and chicken without the skin.
14. If you miss the potato chip crunch, choose cauliflower, broccoli, peppers, carrots, celery, baked chips, saltines, or matzos.
15. Beware of chef salads and Caesar salad.
16. If you are hungry, start your meal with a non-fat soup.
17. Schedule a reasonable after-dinner mini-meal instead of succumbing to an uncontrolled binge.
18. Don't eat fewer than one thousand calories each day.
19. To lose fat do one or more of the following: Eat slightly smaller portions of a balanced diet, cut down on fats, exercise more, eat fewer total calories, stop nibbling after dinner.

CHAPTER 6

Conclusion

6.1 Putting It All Together

Martial arts training, whatever the style, is one of the best things you can do for your body and mind. No matter what your training goals—from future Olympian to weekend warrior—you can get more from your training if you emphasize the following four basics:

1. **Flexibility**—Practice your stretching exercises before and after each martial arts training session. The stretching exercises in this book are specifically designed to increase upper and lower body flexibility.

2. **Strength**—The strength of your legs and torso will be progressively improved by practicing the various isometric stances in chapter two. Each stance requires you to bend your knees while keeping your back erect so the weight of your upper body acts as resistance to your hips, quadriceps, and calves. Strengthen your chest, shoulders, back, and arms with dynamic tension exercises and weights.

3. **Endurance**—Mastering your art requires both the aerobic and anaerobic systems. You can get in an aerobic workout by practicing strikes, blocks, stances, stepping, and combinations. For anaerobic workouts, practice forms, sparring, resistance training, or plyometrics. Anaerobics has been shown to burn more calories quicker than long, slow, distance walking or jogging. Therefore martial arts training is an excellent method of weight reduction.

4. **Concentration**—Let your mind become intimately involved with your body during your workouts. You may discover a new sense of discipline and confidence. Make each technique precise, coordinated and based on a concentrated effort to unite your body and mind.

Other Things to Keep In Mind

If you eat huge high-fat meals and forget to drink enough water, you will dehydrate and look like a sumo wrestler. However, if you eat low-fat, high carbohydrate food, drink lots of water, and eat small meals, you will fuel your muscles and starve the fat.

If you get three hours of sleep and stay awake drinking coffee, you will drain your adrenal glands and have a false sense of alertness. However, if you get enough sleep, meditate or pray regularly, and learn to relax, you will be more alert and your energy levels will skyrocket.

If you sit on the couch and the heaviest thing you lift is a pencil, you will lose your muscle tone and slow your metabolism. However, if you move, stretch, and strengthen your muscles, you will be faster, more coordinated, and burn calories more efficiently.

If you don't practice martial arts, you will lose your speed, endurance, and discipline. However, if you punch and kick three times a week, you will maintain your technique, but more importantly you will remain confident.

If you never observe and spar better fighters, you may not improve your technique. However, if you model yourself after elite athletes, you may add variety and explosiveness to your program.

If you think about martial arts only in the training hall, you will not reach your potential. However, if you spend a few minutes, a few times a week imagining yourself performing magnificently, you will. If you never help somebody else with their technique, you may never master the details. However, if you teach someone to punch or kick correctly, you will refine your own technique.

If you don't enjoy your training, you will probably quit. However, if you create excitement in your practice, you may train for a lifetime. If you never concentrate during your training, you are just dancing. However, if you focus on your imaginary opponent, your techniques will work.

If you give fifty percent during training, you can only give fifty percent during performance. However, if you give one hundred percent during training, giving it all for your performance will be natural.

6.2 Ten Tips to Master Your Art

1. **Fear Nothing:** Any threat or obstacle may be perceived as a challenge. When in danger, become master of your art. Face your fears and conquer them.
2. **Be Cool:** Nothing can move you. Rely on your foundation. Have fun, but be in control of your emotions.
3. **Develop Discipline:** Work hard at perfecting your art. Adhere to a daily training schedule. Most martial artists never fulfill their potential. Although physical limitations such as flexibility are somewhat predetermined, many people never come close to their optimum level.

4. No Worries: Do your best. Delete bothersome thoughts from your memory.

5. Concentrate: Whatever you are doing, do it with energy.

6. Try Softer: Physical ability isn't your only ability. Use maximum effort without tension. Combine force with relaxation.

7. Be Flexible: A schedule is great, but don't be a slave to it. Try different routines. Variety can spur your performance.

8. Show Love: Love people, love work, love your art.

9. Be Compassionate: Your art will make you physically strong, so develop a compassionate heart.

10. Be Joyful: Adjust your goals. Even if you never become a champion, be happy in your physical, mental, and spiritual training.

Appendix: Resources for the Martial Arts Athlete

Fitness Workshop Presentation Company
City Workout
1618 Orrington Ave.
Suite 202 Evanston, IL 60201
1-800-545-city

Supplier of Exercise Bands. Good for resistance exercises without dumbbells.
SPRI Products
1684 Barclay Blvd.
Buffalo Grove, IL 60089

A very good martial arts magazine.
Martial Arts Training
24715 Ave. Rockefeller
Santa Clarita, CA 91380-9018

Supplier of dumbbells and other strength building equipment.
PowerBlock
2020 Austin Road
Owatonna, MN 55060
1-800-555-3001

Continuing education credit program for fitness experts. Certified in ACE and ACSM.
Exercise Etc.
2101 North Andrews Ave.
Suite 201
Fort Lauderdale, FL 33311

Suggested Reading

Beaulieu, J. (1981) "Developing a Stretching Program." *Physician and Sports Medicine.* Vol 9. November.

Benson, H. (1993) *The Wellness Book.* New York: Simon & Schuster.

Edman, K. (1979) "The Effect of Stretch on Contracting Skeletal Muscle Cells." *Cross-Bridge Mechanism in Muscular Contraction.* University Park Press. Baltimore

Eichner, E. (1988) "Circadian Timekeepers in Sports." *The Physician and Sportsmedicine.* vol. 16. Number 2.

Hakkinen, K. (1989) "Neuromuscular and Hormonal Adaptations During Strength and Power training." *Journal of Sports Medicine and Physical Fitness.* Vol. 29.

Holt, L. (1970) "Comparative Study of Three Stretching Techniques." *Perceptual and Motor Skills.* Vol. 31.

Leonard, G. (1987) "Mastery." *Esquire.*

Seabourne, T.G. (1986) " Cross Court Training." *Tae Kwon Do Times.* November issue. pg. 68, 69.

Seabourne, T.G. (1986) " Mental Kicks." *Superfit.* Fall issue. pg. 6.

Seabourne, T.G. (1981) "The Effects of Relaxation and Imagery Training on Karate Performance." *Karate Illustrated.* March issue.

Seabourne, T.G., and Herndon, E. (1986) *Self Defense: A Body-Mind Approach.* Gorsuch-Scarisbrick. Scottsdale, Arizona.

Seabourne, T.G. and McLaughlin, C.V. (1989) "Managing Stress While Performing Police Tasks." *Your Virginia State Trooper Magazine.* pg. 78,79.

Seabourne, T.G., and Jackson, A. (1981) "Effects of Visuo-motor Behavior Rehearsal, Relaxation and Imagery on Karate Performance." *Journal of Sport Psychology.* Vol. 3. no. 3.

Seabourne, T.G., Weinberg, R.S., (1985) " Martial Mind Games: Can You Psyche Yourself Into Winning?" *Inside Karate.* March issue.

Seabourne, T.G., Weinberg, R.S., and Jackson, A., (1985) "Effect of Arousal and Relaxation Instructions Prior to the Use of Imagery." *Journal of Sport Behavior.*

Seabourne, T.G., Weinberg, R. (1983) "Mental Practice: Research Shows It May Improve Your Physical Performance." *Kick Illustrated.* September issue. k48667.

Seabourne, T.G., Weinberg, R.S., and Jackson, A. (1983) "Effect of Individualized Practice and Training of Visuo-motor Behavior Rehearsal In Enhancing Karate Performance." *Journal of Sport Behavior.* Vol. 7. No. 2. pgs. 58-67.

Seabourne, T.G., Weinberg, R.S., and Jackson, A. (1985) "The Effects of Guided VMBR vs. Individualized VMBR Training on Karate Performance." *Karate Illustrated.*

Seabourne, T.G., Weinberg, R.S., Jackson, A., Suinn, R., (1985) "Effect of Individualized, Nonindividualized, and Packaged Intervention Strategies on Athletic Performance." *Journal of Sport Psychology.* Vol. 7. no. 1.

Town, G. (1980) "The Effect of Rope Skipping Rate on Energy Expenditure of Males and Females." *Medicine and Science in Sports and Exercise.* "

Weinberg, R.S., Seabourne, T.G., and Jackson, A. (1982) "Effects of Visuo-Motor Behavior Rehearsal on State-Trait Anxiety and Performance: Is Practice Important?" *Journal of Sport Behavior* Vol. 5. No. 4. pgs. 209-218.

Wescott, W. (1994) "Why Every Adult Should Strength Train." *Nautilus.* Summer

Wilmore, J., and Costill D. (1994) *Physiology of Sport and Exercise.* Human Kinetics Publishers, Champaign, Il.

Index

BOOKS FROM YMAA

6 HEALING MOVEMENTS
101 REFLECTIONS ON TAI CHI CHUAN
A WOMAN'S QIGONG GUIDE
ADVANCING IN TAE KWON DO
ANCIENT CHINESE WEAPONS
ANALYSIS OF SHAOLIN CHIN NA 2ND ED.
ARTHRITIS RELIEF: CHINESE QIGONG FOR HEALING & PREVENTION,
    3RD ED.
BACK PAIN RELIEF: CHINESE QIGONG FOR HEALING & PREVENTION
    2ND ED
BAGUAZHANG
CARDIO KICKBOXING ELITE
CHIN NA IN GROUND FIGHTING
CHINESE FAST WRESTLING: THE ART OF SAN SHOU KUAI JIAO
CHINESE FITNESS: A MIND / BODY APPROACH
CHINESE TUI NA MASSAGE
COMPLETE CARDIOKICKBOXING
COMPREHENSIVE APPLICATIONS OF SHAOLIN CHIN NA
CONFLICT COMMUNICATION
DUKKHA: A SAM REEVES MARTIAL ARTS THRILLER
DUKKHA REVERB: A SAM REEVES MARTIAL ARTS THRILLER
DUKKHA UNLOADED: A SAM REEVES MARTIAL ARTS THRILLER
EIGHT SIMPLE QIGONG EXERCISES FOR HEALTH, 2ND ED.
ENZAN: THE FAR MOUNTAIN
ESSENCE OF SHAOLIN WHITE CRANE
ESSENCE OF TAIJI QIGONG, 2ND ED.
FACING VIOLENCE
FIGHTING ARTS
INSIDE TAI CHI
KATA AND THE TRANSMISSION OF KNOWLEDGE
LITTLE BLACK BOOK OF VIOLENCE
LIUHEBAFA FIVE CHARACTER SECRETS
MARTIAL ARTS ATHLETE
MARTIAL ARTS INSTRUCTION
MARTIAL WAY AND ITS VIRTUES
MEDITATIONS ON VIOLENCE
MIND/BODY FITNESS: A MIND / BODY APPROACH
THE MIND INSIDE TAI CHI
MUGAI RYU: THE CLASSICAL SAMURAI ART OF DRAWING THE SWORD
NATURAL HEALING WITH QIGONG: THERAPEUTIC QIGONG
NORTHERN SHAOLIN SWORD, 2ND ED.
OKINAWA'S COMPLETE KARATE SYSTEM: ISSHIN RYU

PRINCIPLES OF TRADITIONAL CHINESE MEDICINE
QIGONG FOR HEALTH & MARTIAL ARTS 2ND ED.
QIGONG FOR LIVING
QIGONG FOR TREATING COMMON AILMENTS
QIGONG MASSAGE —FUNDAMENTAL TECHNIQUES FOR HEALTH AND
    RELAXATION, 2ND ED.
QIGONG MEDITATION: EMBRYONIC BREATHING
QIGONG MEDITATION—SMALL CIRCULATION
QIGONG, THE SECRET OF YOUTH
QUIET TEACHER
ROOT OF CHINESE QIGONG, 2ND ED.
SHIN GI TAI—KARATE TRAINING FOR BODY, MIND, AND SPIRIT
SHIHAN TE: THE BUNKAI OF KATA
SIMPLIFIED TAI CHI CHUAN 24 & 48 POSTURES
SUNRISE TAI CHI
SURVIVING ARMED ASSAULTS
TAE KWON DO: THE KOREAN MARTIAL ART
TAEKWONDO BLACK BELT POOMSAE
TAEKWONDO: A PATH TO EXCELLENCE
TAEKWONDO: ANCIENT WISDOM FOR THE MODERN WARRIOR
TAEKWONDO: DEFENSES AGAINST WEAPONS
TAEKWONDO: SPIRIT AND PRACTICE
TAI CHI BALL QIGONG: FOR HEALTH AND MARTIAL ARTS
TAI CHI BOOK
TAI CHI CHIN NA: THE SEIZING ART OF TAI CHI CHUAN
TAI CHI CHUAN CLASSICAL YANG STYLE (REVISED
    EDITION)
TAI CHI CHUAN MARTIAL APPLICATIONS
TAI CHI CHUAN MARTIAL POWER
TAI CHI CONNECTIONS
TAI CHI DYNAMICS
TAI CHI QIGONG, 3RD ED.
TAI CHI SECRETS OF THE ANCIENT MASTERS
TAI CHI SECRETS OF THE WU & LI STYLES
TAI CHI SECRETS OF THE WU STYLE
TAI CHI SECRETS OF THE YANG STYLE
TAI CHI SWORD: CLASSICAL YANG STYLE
TAIJIQUAN THEORY OF DR. YANG, JWING-MING
TENGU: THE MOUNTAIN GOBLIN, A CONNOR BURKE
    MARTIAL ARTS THRILLER
TRADITIONAL CHINESE HEALTH SECRETS
TRADITIONAL TAEKWONDO
WESTERN HERBS FOR MARTIAL ARTISTS
XINGYIQUAN, 2ND ED.

DVDS FROM YMAA

ANALYSIS OF SHAOLIN CHIN NA
ADVANCED PRACTICAL CHIN NA IN DEPTH
BAGUAZHANG 1,2, & 3 —EMEI BAGUAZHANG
CHEN STYLE TAIJIQUAN
CHIN NA IN DEPTH COURSES 1: 4
CHIN NA IN DEPTH COURSES 5: 8
CHIN NA IN DEPTH COURSES 9: 12
EIGHT SIMPLE QIGONG EXERCISES FOR HEALTH
THE ESSENCE OF TAIJI QIGONG
FIVE ANIMAL SPORTS
INFIGHTING
KNIFE DEFENSE—TRADITIONAL TECHINIQUES AGAINST DAGGER
MERIDIAN QIGONG
NEIGONG FOR MARTIAL ARTS
QIGONG FOR HEALING
QIGONG MASSAGE—FUNDAMENTAL TECHNIQUES FOR HEALTH AND
    RELAXATION
SHAOLIN KUNG FU FUNDAMENTAL TRAINING 1&2
SHAOLIN LONG FIST KUNG FU: BASIC SEQUENCES
SHAOLIN SABER: BASIC SEQUENCES
SHAOLIN STAFF: BASIC SEQUENCES
SHAOLIN WHITE CRANE GONG FU BASIC TRAINING 1&2
SIMPLE QIGONG EXERCISES FOR ARTHRITIS RELIEF
SIMPLE QIGONG EXERCISES FOR BACK PAIN RELIEF
SIMPLIFIED TAI CHI CHUAN

SUNRISE TAI CHI
SUNSET TAI CHI
SWORD—FUNDAMENTAL TRAINING
TAI CHI ENERGY PATTERNS
TAIJI BALL QIGONG COURSES 1&2—16 CIRCLING AND 16 ROTATING
    PATTERNS
TAIJI BALL QIGONG COURSES 3&4—16 PATTERNS OF WRAP-COILING
    & APPLICATIONS
TAIJI MARTIAL APPLICATIONS: 37 POSTURES
TAIJI PUSHING HANDS 1&2—YANG STYLE SINGLE AND DOUBLE
    PUSHING HANDS
TAIJI PUSHING HANDS 3&4—MOVING SINGLE AND DOUBLE PUSH-
    ING HANDS
TAIJI SABER: THE COMPLETE FORM, QIGONG & APPLICATIONS
TAIJI & SHAOLIN STAFF - FUNDAMENTAL TRAINING
TAIJI YIN YANG STICKING HANDS
TAIJIQUAN CLASSICAL YANG STYLE
TAIJI SWORD, CLASSICAL YANG STYLE
UNDERSTANDING QIGONG 1: WHAT IS QI? • HUMAN QI CIRCULATORY
    SYSTEM
UNDERSTANDING QIGONG 2: KEY POINTS • QIGONG BREATHING
UNDERSTANDING QIGONG 3: EMBRYONIC BREATHING
UNDERSTANDING QIGONG 4: FOUR SEASONS QIGONG
UNDERSTANDING QIGONG 5: SMALL CIRCULATION
UNDERSTANDING QIGONG 6: MARTIAL QIGONG BREATHING
WHITE CRANE HARD & SOFT QIGONG
YANG TAI CHI FOR BEGINNERS

---

more products available from...
YMAA Publication Center, Inc. 楊氏東方文化出版中心
1-800-669-8892 • info@ymaa.com • www.ymaa.com